THE
CANCER
CONQUEROR

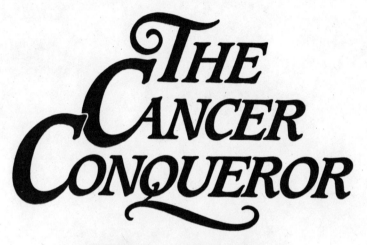

THE
CANCER
CONQUEROR

GREG ANDERSON

WORD PUBLISHING
Dallas · London · Sydney · Singapore

THE CANCER CONQUEROR

LIBRARY OF CONGRESS
Library of Congress Cataloging-in-Publication Data

Anderson, Greg, 1947–
   The cancer conqueror / Greg Anderson.
     p.   cm.
   ISBN 0-8499-0661-X
   1. Cancer—Psychosomatic aspects.   2. Cancer—Psychological aspects. I. Title.
RC262.A66 1988   88–20502
616.99′40019—dc19   CIP

Printed in the United States of America

8 9 8 0 1 2 3 9 RRD 9 8 7 6 5 4 3 2 1

TO
MY WIFE
LINDA
AND
OUR DAUGHTER
ERICA.

Thank you for
your constant
love and support.

You, too, are
CANCER CONQUERORS!

CONTENTS

INTRODUCTION   9

Section 1   THE SEARCH FOR SOLUTIONS   11
Section 2   THE PERSPECTIVE OF PERSONAL
            RESPONSIBILITY   17
Section 3   THE CANCER CONQUEROR
            BELIEVES   27
Section 4   THE CANCER CONQUEROR
            RESOLVES   47
Section 5   THE CANCER CONQUEROR LIVES   79
Section 6   THE CANCER CONQUEROR
            EXPLAINS   117
Section 7   THE CANCER CONQUEROR
            BENEFITS   149

EPILOGUE   155

INTRODUCTION

After my second surgery, the doctors sent me home to die. The lung cancer that they had found four months earlier had now spread to the lymph system. According to statistics I had thirty days to live.

Stunned, it took me about two days to realize I needed help. I needed another plan that was more hopeful than the medical prognosis.

That's when I started a journey that continues to this day. I became determined to seek out people who had lived when they were supposed to die. And having found them, I wanted to find out why they felt they were still alive. And in that process, I hoped I could learn for myself as well.

My experiences have led me to a new respect for the power of the human spirit over illness. In this book, I have tried to distill the principles of conquering cancer and communicate them accurately in a way that will be easy to understand.* There is a message of hope here. This hope can change your life. And in doing so, it just might help add to the length of your life.

Apply the principles you find in *The Cancer Conqueror.* What you believe about getting well, how you handle emotional conflicts, plus the decision to choose joyful living do make a huge difference. Keep your hope alive. You can conquer cancer and perhaps even cure it.

Greg Anderson

* *The Cancer Conqueror* is based on factual experience, but fictional names are used.

SECTION 1

The Search for Solutions

*O*nce there was a man who had just received a diagnosis of cancer.

The man did not want cancer. He wanted to be cured, to be disease-free. He wanted to live a full and happy life.

To him, cancer was a frightening enemy. And the fear it brought was a sinking feeling in his stomach that death was just about to overtake him. Was this all there was to life? There was so much left undone, so much that might have been. Maybe that was the worst part of all.

"Why me?" He had taken care of himself throughout his fifty years. Oh, he didn't always eat exactly the right foods and sometimes didn't get enough sleep. But certainly he never abused his body. Several of his friends were much worse by comparison.

And what did all this mean medically? It was bad enough to think that there might be only a short life ahead. But maybe even worse, maybe a long life of incapacitation. What would that be like?

His mind raced. "How could this happen to me? I'm losing control." It all seemed so frightening, so futile.

In the meantime, the man looked for someone who had already walked the same path, someone who had found the answer and who might be willing to share his or her experience.

First the man began asking the medical team. His family doctor had referred him to a number of medical specialists, but the one person whom the man trusted the most was his oncologist. This particular doctor was highly respected in the community as well as the medical field. He was directing the man's treatment—a plan that included a surgeon, a radiation oncologist, and other professionals.

The man inquired about his chances for successful recovery.

"Excellent," replied the oncologist. "We have every reason to believe that surgery removed the tumor and that chemotherapy will act as a doublecheck."

This was all reassuring. But he still felt a gnawing sense of fear. So many more questions remained unanswered.

He wished he could talk to someone who had been through a similar experience.

Once he found a long-term survivor, but she looked as if she might die any minute. Even though she had survived for five years—the standard "you are cured" time frame—her quality of life was less than desirable. The man wasn't looking for that.

The man knew that for his sake, as well as for the people around him, he had to find his answer soon.

Then he remembered a co-worker who, several years ago, had lived through cancer. And the interesting thing about his friend's experience was that the cancer journey seemed to have changed him—much for the better. Not only was this man's cancer under control, but he was leading a new and better life than ever before.

Maybe I should talk to him right away, thought the man. When he called his friend's home, one of the children said her parents were on a trip and wouldn't return for another three weeks. *Then he certainly must be doing well,* decided the man.

He asked the friend's daughter, "Do you know what doctor your father went to?"

"No," she replied, "I don't know the doctor. But I do know that he spent the most time with the Cancer Conqueror."

"The *Cancer* Conqueror?" asked the man.

"Yes," answered the daughter. "That's the affectionate name we gave to a man and a group of his friends who taught my dad and our family about cancer. We learned that people can conquer cancer and, in doing so, may even cure it."

The man felt a positive, supportive attitude from the girl when she asked, "Do you have cancer?"

"Yes," said the man. "How can I get in touch with the Cancer Conqueror?"

He took down a telephone number, thanked the daughter, and smiled. "How is your father now?" he asked.

"Never been better," said the daughter. "Cancer has changed our whole family's life all for the better."

"Thank you," said the man as he hung up.

This was more than a little strange. Cancer making changes for the better in the life of an entire family? That was a little hard to believe. Yet the daughter sounded so sure. Maybe there was something to be learned from this terrible thing called cancer after all.

The man called the Cancer Conqueror that same morning and they made an appointment for the following afternoon. He couldn't wait to meet the Cancer Conqueror.

SECTION 2

The Perspective of Personal Responsibility

*F*rom the moment the man arrived at the home of the Cancer Conqueror, he felt an excitement and warmth he could not explain. And the feeling was reinforced when the Cancer Conqueror answered the door with a warm greeting and an easy smile.

So this was the Cancer Conqueror! He had such an approachable manner about him. And his smile—it seemed to come as much from his eyes as from his mouth.

The two men made their way to a lovely backyard where some chilled juice had been prepared for them. They pulled up comfortable chairs, and the Cancer Conqueror asked the man to describe briefly his disease and the prognosis.

Then the Cancer Conqueror asked, "Do you have a high level of confidence in your medical team?"

"Yes," said the man, "I believe they are very knowledgeable and that they have the latest in available technology."

"Excellent. The basis for my recovery also started with a fine medical team. I had a great deal of confidence in their abilities and in them as individuals, too. But I insisted that they share all information with me in terms I could understand. And I wanted explanations for each and every test. I had to be part of every treatment decision.

"What I was really doing was taking personal responsibility for my health—personal responsibility for getting well."

"I'm not sure what you mean," said the man. "What *is* personal responsibility for getting well?"

The Cancer Conqueror leaned forward and looked deeply into the man's eyes.

"Personal responsibility for getting well—for conquering cancer—is one of the most important principles in the cancer journey. If you choose this path—the cancer-conqueror path—personal responsibility will come up again and again. It is one of those cornerstone principles that supports everything else.

"Personal responsibility for health means refusing to be a victim. It means participation in recovery by recognizing and changing self-destructive beliefs and behavior. Personal responsibility for health means believing, 'I am in charge of my cancer. My cancer is not in charge of me.'

"And personal responsibility has simple logic to it. The medical team, no matter how esteemed, function largely in the role of mechanics. They are trained in terms of *body*. They can operate and prescribe treatment, but they are not responsible for our life or our health. We are! Nobody can get well for us. We have to do it for ourselves.

"Selecting a medical team that we have a high level of confidence in is perhaps our first responsibility after diagnosis. But once they are in place, our attention must also focus on the role of mind and spirit in this journey."

"Mind and spirit?" asked the man. "I have a physical problem, not an emotional one."

The Cancer Conqueror nodded. His smile said he understood.

"When I encountered cancer, I instinctively knew that

I
Am
In Charge
Of My
Cancer.

My
Cancer
Is Not
In Charge
Of Me.

this was not just an experience on a physical level. I knew that my mind and spirit had a role to play.

"Personal responsibility meant that if I were to live a healthy and full life, whatever the length, that decision rested not with my doctors but with me. I also realized that once my medical team made its contribution, it was my job to discover and use *all* my healing potential. That leads beyond the body to the mind and the spirit."

"Are you saying that cancer is more than just a physical disease?"

"Yes! That's exactly what I'm saying.

"You certainly have a physical problem. It is a problem with your cells. But that's just one facet, one level of the problem. As a person, a living human being, you are much more than your body. You are also your mind and your spirit. That means you can bring these resources as well as the mechanical—the body—to the problem.

"The medical team will do all they can to help the body. If you will support them with good nutrition, exercise, and rest, the body portion of the journey will be in place."

"Okay," said the man. "I'll do those things. But I'm not sure about the mind and the spirit. Can I learn?"

The Cancer Conqueror stopped and smiled. If this person really meant that question, there was hope. With the open attitude of curiosity about the mind and spirit, much could happen. The man stood an excellent chance of being a Cancer Conqueror.

"Come, let's walk," said the Cancer Conqueror. "Let me share some of my personal story."

As they walked to the gate, the man sensed that he was about to hear something special. And he was ready to listen and learn.

"It was lung cancer," said the Cancer Conqueror. "The doctor put his hand on my shoulder and said that surgery

*Cancer
Is More
Than Just
A Physical
Disease.*

was the only answer. The lung would have to come out.

"They performed surgery, but four months later a growth started protruding from my neck. Again, surgery. It was malignant. It had spread throughout the neck and now they could not operate. The surgeon closed the incision, ordered radiation therapy, and told me to get my affairs in order. According to statistics, I had a thirty-day life expectancy."

The man was astonished. "My chances are much better than that. How did you do it?"

The Cancer Conqueror stopped and leaned against the fence.

"After my second surgery, I was frightened and had virtually lost all hope. I believed the doctors' prognosis. The fear of life coming to a sudden end paralyzed me.

"I was sitting on the couch looking at my daughter playing with a doll. I suddenly thought, *I will not live to see her grow up.* It was the lowest point. I don't know of any point of deeper despair. Tears filled my eyes. It was over.

"The next words that came out were full of anger and fear. 'Oh God, what can I do?'

"But somehow through the tears, through the anger and the fear, a different thought came. It was as if someone were saying, 'You may not be given long to live, but *live* as long as you are given.'

"I saw a seed of hope in that thought, a seed that I knew needed special care and attention. It was a seed that provided the framework for me to work through during the countless down times. I knew that every day I had to rededicate myself to living that one day for all it was worth. And this seed is still growing.

"Looking over at my daughter, I thought, *I may not be here to love her tomorrow. But I am here today. How can I show her my love now?*

You May
Not Be
Given Long
To Live,

But Live
As Long
As You
Are Given.

"This is the core of conquering cancer."

"That sounds so simplistic," said the man. "Isn't there more?"

"Much more," agreed the Cancer Conqueror. "This was merely the tip of an enormously powerful discovery. But living for today, doing the best I could to make love my aim, here and now, had a tremendous message of hope for me. It changed not only my health, but my entire life as well. And it can do the same for you.

"If you want to take this journey, your first assignment is to visit three different people over the next three weeks. You will learn about three Cancer Conqueror principles:

Believe
Resolve
Live

"If you complete the assignment, come back and we will talk about why it works and look at the real benefits of conquering cancer.

"Is it something that you would like to do?"

It all seemed so simple, as if there were some sort of formula to use and then everything would be okay.

The man wasn't sure he understood all the Cancer Conqueror had said, but he heard himself saying, "Okay, what do I have to lose?"

The Cancer Conqueror stopped and looked at the man with that now-familiar smile that came from his eyes. "All you have to lose," he said, "are your fears, angers, and guilt. I'll set up the first appointment for you.

"Over the weekend, give thought to your personal responsibility for getting well. YOU ARE IN CHARGE!"

SECTION 3

The Cancer Conqueror Believes

*T*he following Monday, the man found himself at a home just a few blocks from his own. He'd walked by here several times and remembered chuckling at the sign over the doorbell—LOVE SPOKEN HERE.

Now here he was, at this same house seeking answers that he wasn't even sure he knew the questions to. It seemed more than a little ironic.

An attractive woman opened the door. Her voice was pleasant. "Welcome, I'm Mary. I've looked forward to talking with you ever since the Cancer Conqueror called last week. He's quite a person, isn't he?" she asked as she led him to a table where she had hot water and herb teas waiting for them.

"Yes he is," said the man as he sat down. "Do you mind if I take notes?" he asked.

"That's great," said Mary. "When the Cancer Conqueror called, he said for us to cover the area of beliefs. So let's get started.

"The point of departure is to ask you a question. What do you think cancer means?"

"I'm not sure," said the man. "I know it is a serious illness that will probably end my life pretty quickly unless I do something about it. And the Cancer Conqueror said it was more than physical. To me cancer is the worst negative I have ever had to deal with."

Mary smiled. "Those are pretty common beliefs about cancer. Society has conditioned us to think negatively about cancer. And while some of that conditioning can be good, it has resulted in some serious untruths.

"The *three major untruths* we are conditioned to believe about cancer are:

1. Cancer means death.
2. Treatment is ineffective and has bad side effects.
3. Once you contract cancer, there is nothing you can do to help yourself.

"The truths about these statements are:

1. Cancer may or may not mean death.
2. Treatment is getting more effective and side effects less severe every day.
3. Once you contract cancer, there are *many* things you can do—especially spiritually, psychologically, and emotionally—to help yourself.

"The untruths lead to beliefs that result in despair. With despair there is no power. But the truths lead to hope. With hope there is *significant* power.

"What you choose to believe about cancer is crucial to your journey. Note how the truths match three belief areas—the disease itself, the treatment, and your role. Your beliefs about the disease, the treatment, and your role have incredible power over the outcome. You can choose those beliefs."

The man could see why the Cancer Conqueror wanted him to talk to Mary. She was forceful as she talked about beliefs. He actually held most of the negative beliefs Mary talked about.

"I want to believe the hopeful thoughts," admitted

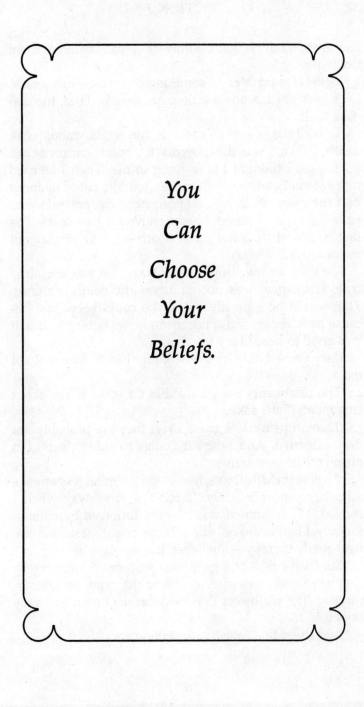

You
Can
Choose
Your
Beliefs.

the man, "but I don't know if I can believe them immediately."

"Beliefs," said Mary, "sometimes don't change easily. Let's look at each one a little more closely. First, the disease itself.

"It really is a fact. Cancer is not synonymous with death. When I was diagnosed with breast cancer seven years ago, I thought I was going to die. Then I learned more about the disease. Cancer is actually cured in about half the cases. And over 80 percent of the patients who have the type of cancer I had survive for five years. The fact is, cancer does not mean death—it may or may not mean death."

The man was writing notes. Okay, that was certainly true. His cancer was not an automatic death sentence. That would be a positive belief he could keep. Just because he had cancer did not mean he was going to die. It was good to hear Mary say that.

Mary paused only long enough for him to have a sip of tea.

"The treatments are next. What do you believe about treatments?" she asked.

The man paused, "I guess I feel they are probably not very effective. And when it comes to side effects, I'm afraid of the possibilities."

Mary seemed to have had a very similar experience with her cancer journey. "I felt the same way when I started. My treatment was surgery followed by chemotherapy. I had heard only bad things about mastectomies. And chemotherapy—I believed it was a last-hope drug.

"But then the doctor gave me assurances. The surgery was more and more effective. And the same for chemotherapy. The truth was that the treatment plan was very hopeful."

"And the side effects?" asked the man.

"I was fortunate," said Mary. "Just as I was beginning the chemotherapy sessions, I read about the psychological component of side effects. Research had tracked a group of people who were given sterile water injections instead of chemotherapy, and a third of them lost their hair anyway."

"I don't understand," said the man.

"The only explanation the researchers could give for the hair loss was psychological in nature. They lost their hair because they *believed* the chemotherapy would do that to them."

"And there is more." Mary continued, allowing no lapse in the conversation. "In another group, 30 percent of the people got sick *on their way* to chemotherapy. They got sick, not after the drug had been administered, not during the administration, but *before*—at the very thought of chemotherapy.

"Of course that doesn't mean no one will ever have side effects again. But it does mean that there is a psychological component in the side effects and that we can work to control that component.

"In short, the belief we want to encourage is that the treatment is our friend. And as our friend, it is effective in helping overcome the physical part of the illness. It is fair to assume, then, that the side effects will, most likely, be very minimal."

"You're asking a lot," said the man. "I'm supposed to start chemotherapy, too. And I don't see those drugs as a friend at all."

Mary continued, "The Cancer Conqueror taught me that as a patient, I needed to believe in my treatment program even more than the physician who prescribed it did! That was a revelation to me. He went on to say that the treatment program was something I needed to get excited about. I would need to align myself with the treatment, believe in its effectiveness, and think of it as a welcome friend. I admit that I spent a lot of time nurturing this one belief."

More notes. The man was starting to see something. The Cancer Conqueror was right. There was more to cancer than just the physical.

"But even more important than beliefs about the disease, the treatment, and the side effects," continued Mary, "are the beliefs we have about our personal responsibility in the cancer journey. The beliefs about our role are very important."

"What do you mean?" asked the man.

"Beliefs are fascinating," said Mary. "For me they started with the thought that my role would be that of the submissive patient. At first I didn't think there was much else I could do.

"Then I was fortunate again. The same library where I found the facts on side effects had more information on other aspects of the cancer experience. Soon I was reading books on the role I could assume with my medical team, with the disease, and with my family. For the first time I was able to exercise some personal control over the illness. I was able to see my role as managing a total treatment program that included my medical team, my mind, and my spirit.

"I studied. I worked. I fanned the flames of my will to live," said Mary with enthusiasm that was contagious. "If there was a book, I read it. If there was a tape, I listened to it. If there was a video, I watched it. And I made notes and summaries of nearly everything on cancer. There is no question in my mind that my self-education was a vital part of the process of getting well.

"Yet as good as all those things were, as important as the self-education process was, I always kept coming back to mind and spirit. It became apparent to me that mind and spirit were the key parts of my treatment plan that were directly under my control.

"It led me to what I consider one of the single most powerful beliefs that I had ever nurtured. I came to see that even though I *had* cancer, I *was not* cancer."

"Whatever do you mean?" asked the man.

Mary smiled as she explained. "I mean to say that by seeing myself not just as my body that was riddled with cancer, but by seeing myself also as my mind and my spirit which were very alive and ready to soar with energy, I was then able to make an important distinction. I was able to separate who I was as a person from what I had as a disease. I had control over my mind and spirit! And my mind and my spirit had cancer only if I allowed it.

"Who I was as a person was much more than what I had as a disease. That's what I mean when I say, 'Even though I have cancer, I am not cancer.' That is a powerful belief."

The man completed his notes. "Tell me more," he said.

"The Cancer Conqueror taught me some other beliefs," said Mary. "One of the most powerful was about the cancer cells themselves. Once I said to the Cancer Conqueror that it was terribly frightening to think of the cancer eating away inside my body. That's when he gently but forcefully corrected this false belief. I remember his words well: 'Cancer cells don't eat other cells. Cancer cells are weak and confused cells.'

"The Cancer Conqueror went on to explain that the cells themselves are not intelligent. They don't make up a bodily organ. Instead, they have gone mad. They are confused."

"That's true," said the man. "I always believed that the cancer was all-powerful. That's a dangerous untruth, isn't it?"

Even
Though
I Have
Cancer,

I Am Not
Cancer.

"Yes," Mary confirmed, "and another important belief puts new perspective on treatment.

"Right in our own bodies is the mortal enemy of cancer cells, our very own immune system. You see, it is not that the surgeons, the radiation, the chemotherapy, or other treatments are all-powerful. They themselves can't cure the cancer. No! The truth is that those treatments help the body's immune system heal itself—from within! The medical team is in a support role to the body's own healing power! Isn't that a revelation?"

The man sat contemplating what he had just heard. This was powerful! And he realized that the truth he was hearing could have a far-reaching impact on his own program for recovery. "Yes," he said, "I think I'm beginning to understand the huge significance of what you just said."

Mary went on, "The Cancer Conqueror taught me that cancer has a significant psychological, emotional, and spiritual component. We can understand more about this part by looking at stress and the way we handle it.

"You'll learn more about stress later. But the essentials are that mismanaged stress can lead to both a physical and psychological reaction that primes the body to respond. This priming is mind-controlled. Either responding inappropriately or suppressing a response can give the body confusing signals. The result is that our own immune systems become depressed and less effective in warding off potential cancer cells.

"These essentials are documented in a field of medicine called psychoneuroimmunology. Very basically, it recognizes that the mind and spirit do affect the body.

"Thoughts of fear, anger, and guilt can lead to sickness on more levels than just the physical. Yet thoughts of love, joy, and peace lead to health and well-being on more than just the physical level."

The man put all this in his notes. Most of what Mary said was new thinking for him.

The man hesitated a moment, "Does this mean I gave myself cancer?"

"No, no!" said Mary. "That's much too rigid a view. You didn't give yourself cancer. However, our inability to handle stress constructively, to resolve conflicts creatively, and to manage anxieties may have contributed to the beginning of illness. Of course, it wasn't a conscious decision. We never set out to give ourselves cancer. But yes, we may have contributed to the onset on a subconscious level.

"Now here is the hopeful part: If you believe that you may have contributed to your illness, then you must also believe that you have the power to contribute to your recovery.

"The psychological and spiritual components can work either for us or against us. The choice is ours."

The man nodded his thoughtful understanding. This belief was starting to make sense. And it was opening a door of hope.

"Perhaps understanding the context will help," Mary added. "Behind all these statements lies a revolutionary assumption that needs to be understood and believed at a deep level. The assumption is this—cancer is a process."

"I'm afraid you'll have to explain that a bit more," said the man.

"Conventional medical wisdom teaches us that cancer is a thing, a spatial entity or physical condition. My doctors talked about cancer as tumors. They talked about cancer as an abnormal state marked by those tumors. To them the word *cancer* was a noun—a thing."

"That is, of course, true," said the man.

"It is," Mary nodded. "But it is also a rather shallow

definition of cancer. For example, I once thought of a golf ball as simply a round, white sphere with dimples in its surface. But that was before I saw a golf ball that had been sliced in half.

"There was the outer white, dimpled shell all right. But there was also much more. Right under the surface was a deep red rubberized coating. This covered and secured the next layer, which was made up of tan-colored rubber bands. They were everywhere, tightly wound all around inside the ball. And in the very center was a hard, black rubber ball about the size of a large pea.

"Now for me to define a golf ball as round, white, and dimpled after having seen the cutaway ball would be incomplete. The same is true for cancer."

"I still don't understand what you are driving at," said the man.

"Just this. Examine your own cancer experience beyond just the surface appearances. Open your mind to the full dimensions of the idea that cancer is more than a physical condition. Cancer is not a disease of which you are a victim. It is a process which you can master.

"The medical community uses cancer as a noun. I encourage you to make cancer into a verb, an action verb! I challenge you to start to think, see, and feel yourself as 'cancering.'"

"*Cancering?*" asked the man.

"Yes," said Mary. "The verb *cancering* shifts our focus away from a disease we have and into the context of a process we are going through."

"Cancering," mused the man. "It has a strange sound to it."

"Good," said Mary. "That strange sound will help remind you that this is a process and that you have an important part in it."

"Will you trace this cancering process?" asked the man.

Cancer

Is Not

A Disease

Of Which

You

Are

A Victim.

It Is

A Process

Which

You Can

Master.

"Okay," said Mary, "let's walk through the typical steps.

"First, we need to understand that not every cancer patient's experience would fit this pattern. Certainly there are genetic causes of cancer. Some people are born with that unfortunate physical predisposition. And there is no question that carcinogens in our environment, in our foods, all around us, can trigger malignancy.

"Even so, there is increasing evidence that many cancers are stress-related. In fact, the percentage may be much higher than first imagined. One group of researchers in a recent study found that more than 90 percent of the participants could trace the onset of cancer to a period of high stress. The researchers went so far as to say that, in their opinion, this same percentage probably applied to nearly all cancers."

"Astounding," said the man.

"The evidence is becoming overwhelming. Many times the body will start cancering because of the prolonged emotional conflict that has its base in stress. And this emotional conflict—the feelings of loss, hopelessness, and despair—can lead to mental depression. Today scientists feel that there must be some sort of direct link between mental depression and immune system depression. The result can be the onset of disease.

"Now we need to make a careful distinction. This is not to say that all people who are having emotional distress will start cancering. No, it is to say that the cancering process often begins on the emotional level.

"Perhaps the first symptoms are barely detectable. And it may be months, even years, before physical symptoms occur. The physical symptoms eventually compel the patient to seek a medical diagnosis and a treatment plan is then developed and begun.

"And while a proper treatment program on the physical

level is mandatory, I encourage you to understand that the cancering process is far more inclusive. The physical portion—the tumor—is only a signal in the process."

The man sat silently for a moment. "My intuition accepts this. But my rational mind wants to resist it."

Mary said, "Are you assuming that cancering excludes the traditional, rational, medical approach? Cancering includes it. We are simply opening our minds to go beyond the limits of that thinking. Because the truth is, cancering is both rational and intuitive.

"Believe it, cancer doesn't just happen to us. It can spring from inner disharmony, either physical or emotional. And this has two implications. One is responsibility. We may have been responsible, at least subconsciously, for contributing to the onset of the illness.

"But the second implication is opportunity. Cancer is a reversible disease, and there are patients who happily experience reversal every day.

"Our task is to choose harmony at the level of the mind and the spirit. Only then can we help our bodies regenerate and achieve physical harmony.

"This is truly conquering cancer. And in conquering, we might even cure it."

Mary continued, "The Cancer Conqueror likes to help us reframe the meaning of cancer. By reframing, he means looking at the illness in a different light.

"And while this perspective includes new ways to consider several beliefs about the illness, the treatment, and our roles, the Cancer Conqueror encourages the primary belief that *cancer is a message to change.*

"Yes, cancer does have a physical component. And yes, it can be life-threatening. But even though this is true, cancer is foremost a warning for us to change.

"The Cancer Conqueror calls this change *resolve.* When we resolve those areas in our lives where there is unrest,

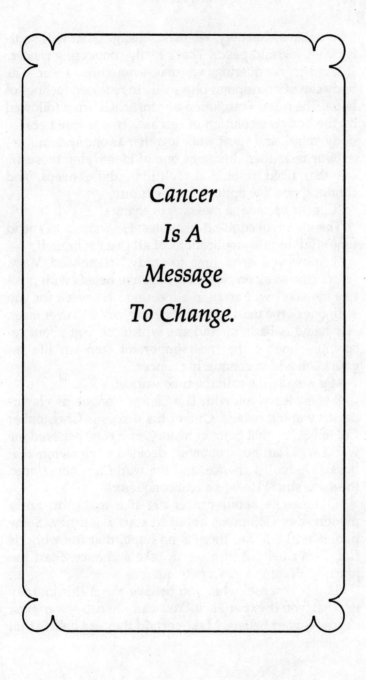

Cancer
Is A
Message
To Change.

where there is anxiety, we make changes that will nour-ish love, joy, and peace. That's really conquering cancer.

"And in conquering, we may even cure cancer. The body can often respond physically to renewed feelings of hope. The mind's resolution of conflicts is often followed by the body's resolution of disease. This is true because body, mind, and spirit work together as one system.

"Our task, then, becomes one of identifying those ar-eas that need resolution, fulfilling those needs, and choosing positive options for the future.

"Cancer becomes a message to change."

The man looked at all his notes. He wanted to spend time studying the implications of all this for himself.

"I know you need time to study," responded Mary. "Work this week on replacing negative beliefs with posi-tive beliefs. I will arrange a meeting next week for you with one of the most beautiful people you will ever meet. Her name is Barbara, and she will teach you about re-solving—one of the most important steps in life re-education and in conquering cancer."

Mary made the call; the time was set.

"Let me leave you with The Cancer Conqueror's favor-ite story about beliefs. One of his heroes is Christopher Columbus. At that point in history, everyone believed the world was flat. But Columbus decided to challenge that belief. He took a chance, and the world has never been the same since! He was a real conqueror!

"Our beliefs about cancer are like that. You are a modern-day Columbus about to start a journey. Some people will tell you there is no hope, that the world is flat. Don't believe it! Instead, take a chance. Start the journey. Become a cancer conqueror!

"In a real sense, what you believe about this journey is what you'll experience. You can choose—you *must* choose—your beliefs. Make certain they are beliefs that serve you well. Will those beliefs instill despair or will they inspire hope? You choose."

The man left, touched by Mary's power and authority. He was so impressed that he stopped his car down the block, got out his notebook, and made a summary of the positive beliefs right there.

POSITIVE BELIEFS SUMMARY

THE ILLNESS
1. I do not believe cancer is synonymous with death.
2. I believe cancer cells are weak and confused; they don't eat other cells.

THE TREATMENT
3. I believe treatment is very effective against these weak and confused cells.
4. I believe the side effects, if any, can be controlled.
5. I believe my own immune system overcomes cancer cells daily.

MY ROLE
6. I believe I am personally responsible for my cancer journey.
7. I believe I manage my total treatment program.
8. I believe I am "cancering." It is a process I can master.
9. I believe I can control the emotional, psychological, and spiritual aspects of the illness.
10. I believe cancer is a message for me to change.

SECTION 4

The Cancer Conqueror Resolves

*E*arly the following week, the man was at the door of Barbara's home. The first thing he noticed about Barbara was her smile. It was that same kind of joyful expression he had seen in Mary and in the Cancer Conqueror. And Barbara's voice—it was calm and soothing, another indication of her obvious warmth. They made their way to the patio.

"How is your journey progressing?" began Barbara.

"Well, I've just started," replied the man. "But already the difference in my beliefs is significant. I'm less frightened of the disease. And I also feel more confident in my treatment and in my medical team."

"Excellent," said Barbara. "And where are you in terms of your role?"

"My role is the area that confuses me most. Frankly, I really doubt that what I think or feel will have much effect on the cancer. So I'm not sure about my role."

"Let's discuss that," said Barbara. "The Cancer Conqueror teaches us that much of our role is in the area he calls *'resolve.'*

"Resolve starts with some real basics—diet and exercise. Good nutrition is essential for wellness. Information on sensible eating habits is available from a variety of sources. Seek this information out. Contact the National Cancer Institute for their guidelines. Consider nutritional

49

supplements. Become your own nutrition expert. Act on the belief that what you put in your body is important. You deserve the best in nutrition.

"And exercise. Many people have significant issues to resolve here. Even patients with limiting conditions can maintain an exercise program to some degree. The benefits are both physical and psychological. The type of exercise and the frequency are up to you. The Cancer Conqueror personally uses a half hour three times a week as his yardstick. I have done the same and have chosen walking. Like your research in the area of nutrition, study the literature and become your own exercise expert. Remember, the goal here is to feel more energized, not to become a super athlete.

"But as important as diet and exercise are, when the Cancer Conqueror talks about resolve, he is really putting his emphasis on issues of a psychological and emotional nature. In fact, he is really starting at the point of loving ourselves. Unless we have a healthy respect for ourselves, we probably won't eat right or exercise.

"Resolve goes much deeper than the externals of diet and exercise. When we examine the issue of resolve, we are really focusing on identifying and clearing our lives of emotional roadblocks and self-destructive behavior. This is very important because the resolve principle is based on the premise that emotions affect us physically."

"Is that really provable?" asked the man.

"I'm not certain what you require in terms of proof," continued Barbara. "The whole area of psychoneuroimmunology, or PNI for short, is documenting this mind over illness phenomenon. And it is for real. I encourage you to be open to the possibilities in it.

"Simply stated, the Cancer Conqueror encourages us to acknowledge that attitudes, beliefs, and thoughts go together to create a mental and emotional outlook toward

Beliefs,

Attitudes,

And

Feelings

Lead To

Illness

Or

Wellness.

life, an emotional lifestyle. Those emotions, either positive or negative, translate to the physical. Our beliefs, attitudes, and feelings lead to illness or wellness.

"Perhaps even more astounding, the Cancer Conqueror
teaches us that emotions can play a central role in cancer's
onset and course."

"Wait," interrupted the man. "You're saying things that
aren't really proven. I'm a businessman. I need proof.
Anyway, I thought we were going to talk about resolve,
not emotions."

Barbara observed his surprising resistance. How could
she break through? Could his reaction be a clue to his
problem?

While it wasn't Barbara's style to be confrontive, she
heard herself firmly telling the man, "Listen, please listen
with your mind; don't just hear with your ears."

The man stared at her. It wasn't hard to sense his
discomfort. Or was it thinly disguised anger?

"We *are* talking about resolve," continued Barbara. "But
emotions are the issue at the very core of resolve.

"I am not a medical doctor or researcher. However,
PNI experts have given us much evidence that emotions
occupy a central role in health. Consider this:

Cancer cells are regularly present in virtually all
people. Yet relatively few of these people become ill.
That is because the body's immune system is so powerful. It is the natural enemy of abnormal cells. The
immune system routinely contains or destroys these
cells, allowing them to be carried away through natural bodily processes.

"Yet, when a malignant cell is not destroyed, what is
the reason behind the immune system's not working?

What lapse in the body's defenses might allow these cells to develop into a life-threatening tumor? Why has it developed now? What may have caused the immune system to function at less than full capacity when for years it did operate so very effectively?

"Some people answer this by insisting it is a matter of genetics. Others say diet. Still others teach that it is carcinogens in the environment.

"All these may have a contribution to make in answering the question, 'Why cancer now?' But none offers a full explanation."

Barbara leaned forward and touched the man's arm. "Listen very carefully," she said. "This is perhaps as close as I will get to offering you the proof you seem to need."

The man sat quietly. Barbara continued:

"Genetics, carcinogens, and diet do play a role in the development of cancer. But why aren't they consistently the trigger? If there is genetic predisposition to cancer, it has always been there. Diet may play a part, but in all likelihood, the patient's diet has actually been rather predictable for years. And what about carcinogens? Most people have certainly been exposed to harmful substances before. So why now? What is different at this point in time that would allow the cancer to develop?

"It is at this point that PNI brings us back to the emotional components. What is different? Early research has demonstrated that the development of cancer requires more than just the presence of abnormal cells; it requires also a suppression of the body's natural defenses, the immune system.

"And the difference that could suppress the immune system? Changed emotional states."

The man was listening intently.

"Not only *changed* emotional states, but *charged* emotional states. Fear. Anger. Guilt. All negative emotional states. All commonly the result of mismanaged stress. All potentially capable of depressing the person and the immune system."

The man was starting to write some notes now. Barbara glanced down to see him circle the word *stress*.

"Much of the emotional side of cancer," continued Barbara, "can be understood in the framework of stress. Actually, the issue isn't the stress, but how we manage that stress."

"Tell me more," said the man.

"There are times that each of us faces highly stressful situations, when major emotional upsets seem to dominate our lives. For years the medical community has documented that illness is more likely to occur following highly stressful events in people's lives.

"Some illnesses and their link to stress are readily accepted by the medical community—ulcers, high blood pressure, headaches, even some heart disease. More recently, though, backaches, infections, and even accidents have been seen to increase when the person is dealing with emotional upset. Do you believe all this is true?"

"Yes," agreed the man.

"Good," said Barbara. "It *is* true. And research is finding more and more diseases that are linked to stress all the time.

"Stress can translate to changes in emotional states. Stress can challenge the way we relate to life. Perhaps it challenges our habits, relationships, or our self-image. We 'feel' these challenges—emotionally."

"Is this like the 'fight or flight' response?" asked the man.

"That's exactly it. The human body is endowed with some fantastic capabilities that protect us. When our early ancestors encountered a tiger in their path, there was an immediate reaction. Their breathing speeded up, their adrenaline flowed, and their heart beat faster. When presented with a stressful situation, the body prepared the person either to stay and battle the tiger or to get away from the area as quickly as possible. Thus, the fight or flight response.

"Now most twentieth century people don't normally have to deal with a wild animal in their path. But we do have to deal with mental tigers—all the time. And those are the stresses that can trigger the same bodily reactions.

"Instead of fighting or fleeing, which actually puts to use adrenaline, rapid heartbeat, and faster breathing, modern-day people often suppress or even deny their response. The body's response to an emotional reaction does not get discharged. When we have no outward action available, the stress is internalized. And internalized stress can set us up for trouble.

"It's amazing. Research has found that stress is related to both negative and positive change. While an event like the death of a spouse ranks at the very top of the chart and is certainly negative, a normally positive event such as marriage also produces significant stress. The point is that both negative and positive events of life require new coping skills. Both can often be experienced as emotional conflict.

"It is not enough merely to analyze the stressful events or acquire the new coping skills. We must move to the emotions behind the stress that invariably have their roots in some form of fear, anger, or guilt."

The man was taking many notes by now.

"Then the key point becomes how we manage the emotions associated with stress. Two things must happen in successful stress management. The Cancer Conqueror calls this management the StresSolverSystem:

CHANGE YOUR PERCEPTION OF YOURSELF
AND
CHANGE YOUR PERCEPTION OF YOUR PROBLEM!

"It is really that basic. We need to change our perception of ourselves and our ability to handle whatever life problems face us, particularly the problems prior to cancer. Plus, we need to be able to perceive actual personal problems as being less threatening. Arguably, you could solve the emotional conflict with just one change in perception. But the StresSolverSystem of increasing personal power and decreasing problem power is the essence of successful stress management."

More notes. Was she breaking through?

"The outcome of mismanaged stress is, predictably, emotional conflict. And the outcome of continuing emotional conflict—chronic fear, anger, and guilt—can lead to feelings of helplessness, hopelessness, and despair. From here, it is a short step to depression."

"Okay," said the man. "But this doesn't necessarily mean I'll get cancer."

"That's correct," said Barbara. "There is no 100 percent fixed link. But PNI studies are demonstrating there is some correlation between a depressed mind and a depressed immune system."

"How is that?" pursued the man.

"The heart of the immune system is the person's white blood cells. In an amazing discovery recently, white blood cells were shown to have neuroreceptors. This means that feelings, our emotions, may be biochemically transmitted to and 'felt' by the immune system. This is significant.

StresSolverSystem

Change Your
Perception
Of Yourself
And

Change Your
Perception
Of Your
Problem.

"Just as negative and positive emotions can and do affect the human spirit, they also would seem to affect the immune system. And a chronically depressed immune system can lead to illnesses of many kinds, including cancer.

"Mind affecting body and emotions directing, or maybe even controlling, health make perfect sense. When you have previously been ill, didn't that make you feel psychologically down? In that case, body affected mind. It follows that the reverse could also be true, that mind can affect body. PNI is proving that even as we speak. This is much more than theory."

The man looked thoughtful, pondering what Barbara was saying. "It fits my case," he said. "I lost my job about a year ago. I've tried everything I can think of, but there is nothing I can do to get suitable work. It makes me so mad. I just hate my old boss. And I feel so worthless. I'm really depressed."

Barbara realized now what the problem was. What the man said gave her some of the insight she needed to assist him in resolving his particular situation. Realizing that this was a delicate task of self-discovery, she proceeded gently but firmly.

"I think I can understand how you feel. It has to be tough. But let's stop for a moment and apply what I've just said. Like it or not, losing a job doesn't make you angry. . . . *You* make you angry. Being fired doesn't make you feel worthless. . . . *You* make you feel worthless. You choose those feelings.

"Feelings of helplessness and hopelessness," said Barbara, "were at the heart of the development of my cancer. Let me share my experience. In many ways it parallels yours.

"After thirty-two years of marriage and four wonderful children, my husband and I were divorced. With no small amount of self-pity, I described it by saying, 'He just left me.' I felt fearful, angry, and worthless. Then I became depressed. I viewed myself as a victim."

"A victim under your husband's control, or just a victim out of control?" asked the man.

"Actually both," said Barbara. "And I even took it a step further. I saw myself as a victim of life. What I mean is that I let the crisis situation of the divorce touch all areas of my life. I suppose my reasoning was something like, *If I am a failure as a wife and mother, I must be a failure at everything else.* Mentally and emotionally, I took everything to its worst possible conclusion.

"I then reasoned, *If I am a failure, personally helpless in all life's areas, my life is hopeless. I am a victim of whatever life decides to serve me; a victim with a capital V.*

"I failed to realize hope and hopelessness are both a choice. And I have a personal responsibility for those choices! Why not choose hope?

"The Cancer Conqueror is currently trying to help a friend who was recently diagnosed with prostate cancer. This man adopted a victim stance that included a belief that cancer was a virtual death sentence and that he would probably become impotent as a result of treatments. This man sees himself as being trapped by events beyond his control. He views himself as having no meaningful way to deal with these issues. He is filled with despair. He has chosen an emotional outlook that recognizes only helplessness. He's become a victim to what life has given him. He has surrendered his power and personal responsibility to choose hope. This is the classic victim stance."

"That's a very descriptive illustration," replied the man. "This victim stance seems to relate to my own situation of being out of work and developing cancer, doesn't it?"

"It might," said Barbara. "You be the judge of that." She

Hope
And
Hopelessness
Are Both
A Choice.

Why
Not Choose
Hope?

was encouraged. The man was at least acknowledging the possible link between his emotional state and cancer. Barbara would carefully help him take the next step.

"For me," continued Barbara, "the victim stance actually started with my self-image, including what I was supposed to do in life. It is a typical pattern the Cancer Conqueror describes like this:

1. *A series of high-stress events tears at the person's self-image.* I am faced with divorce. My self-talk based on my self-image says, "I am 'supposed' to be married. Early in my life, I was taught that marriage and motherhood meant success. Now that I am divorced, I must be a failure."

2. *The person's self-allowed techniques for coping are inadequate in response to the self-image threat.* My self-talk says, "Life for me was 'supposed' to be as a wife and mother. I have no idea how a divorced person is 'supposed' to function. I am not in control."

3. *The person sees no way to resolve his or her emotional needs and becomes a victim.* Self-talk speaks out again, "I can't go on. The situation is hopeless. *I* am helpless."

Barbara continued, "While my divorce is a rather obvious example, all of us adopt victim stances. A person in a dead-end job is afraid to move. An abused wife is fearful of leaving an abusive mate. Even attitudes like 'That's just the way I am,' use the victim stance as a convenient way to avoid personal change and growth. In fact, we can choose to be victors instead of victims!"

"This really does relate to my being out of work," said the man. "I once viewed myself as being productive and successful. That became my self-image. That was *me!* When I was dismissed—I just hate to use the word 'fired'—my whole reason for living ceased to exist. And I was defenseless. There was nothing I could do. I felt powerless. Life became unmanageable. And anger ruled

We Can

Choose

To Be

Victors

Instead Of

Victims!

to the point of rage. I was, and I guess I feel I still am,
that victim. I sometimes feel so out of control."

Wow, Barbara thought to herself, *this could be a turning
point! He has opened his mind to renewal.* The man's words
had come fast and with such emotional force. This was
excellent!

She spoke ever-so-sensitively, "You have just taken
what is perhaps the most difficult step in conquering
cancer. None of us wants to concede weakness or helplessness. But by doing so, you have opened yourself to
wonderful possibilities. You can transform this attitude
into self-renewal."

The two sat silently for several moments.

"But what do I do?" continued the man. "I still feel so
vulnerable. It's terrifying!"

Vulnerable didn't come close to describing how he really felt. He was emotionally naked. He had bared his
soul to a virtual stranger. He didn't even talk to his wife
about some of these feelings. It was frightening to be
so open. He realized Barbara was answering his question, and he struggled to focus his mind on what she was
saying.

"What you do now is begin to work on renewing your
mind and your emotions. The victim stance is full of fears,
angers, and guilts. *They* are what you'll work on first.
That is what conquering cancer is all about, taking personal responsibility for changing our negative emotions."

The man was reflective as he tried hard to understand
some of the implications of what Barbara was telling him.

"I'm not good at expressing my emotions," admitted
the man. "I have always believed that some feelings were
best left unsaid. In fact, my father always said that people who talk about them seem pretty weak."

"Interesting that you should say that," said Barbara.
"The Cancer Conqueror helped me so much when he

shared the three most consistent traits of the cancer-prone personality:

"First, the typical cancer personality has a tendency to **bottle up emotions**. You've just shared your thoughts on how you express your feelings as 'best left unsaid.' In my case," continued Barbara, "I tended to play 'poor me' and go into a prolonged silence."

The man chuckled. "I've done some of that."

"We all have," said Barbara. "And it is related to the second tendency, excessive **difficulty grieving loss**. In my divorce, I felt as if I had been done the ultimate wrong. I felt abandoned by my husband. And when the children wouldn't take my side, I felt totally unappreciated. It was an overwhelming sense of loss. And I continued living with those feelings until the Cancer Conqueror began to work with me on expressing my grief over those losses."

The man responded, "I've never thought of my job loss in terms of grief. I suppose that is one framework in which to analyze it, though. I do know it has been a very difficult year. And I feel profoundly empty. I suppose some mourning is taking place inside."

Barbara nodded her agreement; she was encouraged. The man was trying. He was working at this very sensitive assignment. And he was making progress. She continued:

"The third most common characteristic of a typical cancer profile is **judgmentalism**, being unduly critical of others. No question—I certainly did that, particularly where it concerned my husband. In fact, I'm ashamed to say that I really went through life being critical of others. It was a twisted attempt to pull myself up by pushing others down."

The man was contemplative. "I suppose I carry some of all three personality traits."

"Perhaps," said Barbara. "Those personality character-
istics can lead to fear, anger, and guilt that can depress
the immune system and allow cancer, and other illnesses,
to flourish."

"Here we are again. I keep thinking I caused my own
cancer!" sighed the man.

"Recall our beliefs?" asked Barbara. "Just remember
that we probably did contribute to the illness on a subconscious level.

"But the real key is this: If you acknowledge that you
may have contributed to the illness, then, by definition,
you must also acknowledge that you have the ability to
contribute to your wellness."

"I do remember," said the man. "I need to find out how
I contributed negatively. Then it follows that I can reverse it and contribute to health positively."

"Exactly! Excellent!" said Barbara. "Remember, cancer
is a reversible disease. You can contribute to that reversal."

"That's powerful!" said the man.

The man thought, *This is simple yet so profound. On an
intuitive level, the mind-affects-body principles make sense.
And if science can't accurately explain electricity, yet em-
braces it, why do I demand a full explanation of psychoneuroimmunology? I want to reverse my disease. I want LIFE!*

"Okay," said the man. "I want to get well! I'm choosing
life! Where do I start to resolve?"

Barbara beamed! *Choosing life!* Those words affirming
the will to live were powerful. Perhaps he had turned the
corner in his thinking.

"You've already started," smiled Barbara. "What you
do next is take a rigorous emotional inventory of yourself.
The Cancer Conqueror gives us three questions that, if
treated with seriousness, will lead us to higher self-
awareness. You'll want to take notes here.

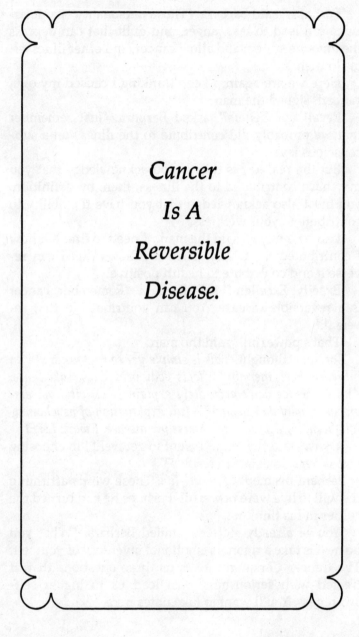

Cancer
Is A
Reversible
Disease.

"First, ask yourself **what high-stress, emotionally disruptive events happened to you in the year or two prior to diagnosis?** This is the stress-management issue. High-stress events can be identified in many patients. But what the Cancer Conqueror really wants us to do is get in touch with the way we reacted to those events. Did we respond to the events with paralyzing fear? Or did we get angry and let anger turn to smoldering resentment? Or did guilt cause such a sense of shame that we may have felt we deserved some kind of punishment? And given the perspective of time, can we now look at different and more constructive ways of handling the situation?

"Second, **what emotional needs might you be meeting or masking with the cancer?**"

"What do you mean?" asked the man.

"Just this. Cancer gets you cards and get well wishes from friends and relatives. It can certainly get you out of work. You can stay at home in bed. It gets you attention, no small amount of sympathy, and may even serve as a means of obtaining nurturing from an otherwise nonnurturing spouse. Just think of that power!

"Cancer is a great permission-giver, allowing both patient and family an acceptable reason to say no to the demands of others. It can also provide a reason to say yes to things that have been put off or otherwise neglected in a person's life."

"I've never really thought about cancer that way before," said the man.

"The Cancer Conqueror," continued Barbara, "calls these cancer games. His real point is to get us to look at the motivation behind our illness-related behavior. It is a fact—in our society sickness is a very powerful force, one that is often rewarded. Patients can manipulate that force, misusing it to meet their needs. Some people emotionaliy cling to the disease. It's their newfound way of fulfilling emotional needs that otherwise have gone unmet."

"That seems incredible to me," said the man.

"Incredible but true," said Barbara. "You will be invited to join a group of us who meet regularly. There you will meet a woman who not only has cancer, but in her lifetime has had nine elective surgeries, currently takes eleven different prescriptive medications, and claims this is the best she has felt in twenty-five years!

"She may be feeling better now than at anytime in the last twenty-five years, but the fact that she still recounts her many illnesses over and over again is a give-away that she probably is manipulating her disease. It's her best way of getting love and even some attention from her otherwise angry and resentful husband.

"The Cancer Conqueror brings us back again and again to this point of examining what needs we might be meeting or masking with the illness. 'Why do I need this illness?' and 'What am I gaining from this illness?' become important issues for us to understand fully. I encourage you to spend all the time you need here.

"This leads to the third question, **what healthy options might you choose to fulfill these needs?** Emotional needs are real. Denying them has probably been part of our problem. The Cancer Conqueror encourages us to recognize the real needs that we feel; he encourages us to look at them squarely and not deny them. He also gives us permission to fulfill those needs but encourages us to do it in a positive, healthy way."

"In the next step of your journey, you'll study LIVE. The whole thrust there is to suggest positive ways, indeed a whole healthy lifestyle, that will meet these needs and contribute to your total wellness.

"But first, let's complete this issue of resolve. Here is an important point. I give you permission to give yourself permission to make certain your needs are met! What do you suppose is your number one need?"

"Mine is simple. I need a job," said the man.

"Wait," said Barbara persuasively. "Look more deeply than that. What are you really after?"

"What do you mean?" he asked.

"Let me offer some examples. In my case," continued Barbara, "I felt I needed to be married. Then the Cancer Conqueror helped me see that what I was really after was feeling loved. But I was going about achieving that goal in a strange and self-destructive way. I was measuring the fulfillment of my love needs by the amount of attention and affection I received.

"When I did that, I always set myself up for disappointment; my husband and children could satisfy those needs only for short periods of time. And when I didn't receive attention and affection, I doubted my self-worth and began to fear being rejected and abandoned. In my search for emotional fulfillment, I manipulated the people most dear to me and caused them to resent me. In some ways, I can understand why my husband left even after all those years we had together.

"The Cancer Conqueror helped me resolve nearly all those issues when he said that my job was to forgive—myself and others. Then he traced how certain processes help people release resentments and forgive both real and perceived wrongs, thus opening the mind and the body to healing. In fact, the Cancer Conqueror believes this is an essential part in getting well.

"Forgiveness was a breakthrough issue for me. It was the process of letting go of the thoughts I had harbored about people who I perceived were harming me. It was equally a process of letting go of the thoughts I had kept about my harming others.

"I no longer saw myself as always being right and

My Job
Is To
Forgive —
Myself
And
Others.

others as always being wrong. I was not innocent and others guilty. That thinking had put me into the blame game where I was seeing myself as a victim, not responsible for my own emotional choices. I was surrendering that power over myself to others. What a mistake! Now I could choose differently. Now I could look upon myself and others with love.

"In fact, for the first time I realized others were doing the best they could, given their level of awareness. And that applied to me as well. The issue was not blame at all.

"I remember one exercise that was most helpful. The Cancer Conqueror had us write out a blame list. We wrote out individuals names, and next to it what we blamed them for. Interestingly, the first name on the list had to be our own. Then, in a joyful ceremony, we all crumpled our lists up in a ball and threw them in a trash can. Then we took the trash cans outside and burned the lists. It was marvelous! It is an event that is vividly etched in my memory, and to this day, it helps me to stop blaming and start forgiving.

"Forgiveness became an important vehicle—a major tool for me to use in the resolve process. I actively forgave others. In fact, I wished them well and imagined good things happening to them. It was really wonderful. And I forgave myself. I realized I could feel loved whether I was married or single, whether my children sided with me or my husband. I realized that my feeling loved was not dependent on others showing me attention or affection. It was instead dependent upon my showing love to others. Whenever I did, I felt loved. And I believe that by resolving this emotional conflict, I helped my body heal itself. Does that make sense? Does that fit you?" asked Barbara.

"I'm not sure," pondered the man quietly.

"For me," Barbara went on, "the real need was to

replace fear, anger, and guilt with love, joy, and peace. 'Being married' and 'needing to feel loved' were only symptoms of a deeper need. Perhaps that is what you're really after.

"Time after time the people who conquer cancer are the ones who work systematically at resolving their emotional conflicts. The main issues are accepting personal responsibility on all levels of life, frank examination of fundamental beliefs, better management of stress, improving self-image, and nurturing better relationships through loving and forgiving. There's more, but that's the heart of it.

"I believe a cancer conqueror needs to get to the point where he or she says, 'I value myself and I am unwilling to remain miserable. I will no longer live life this old destructive way. I will change.'"

The man was thoughtful as he finished his notes, *". . . unwilling to remain miserable; . . . a new person."*

"Your experience of extended unemployment is common. I'm thinking of a man who is part of our Cancer Conqueror group who was also fired from his job. He was a senior officer in one of the largest companies in this city. In fact, his departure was carried in the newspapers. He felt disgraced. His entire self-image was centered around his job. And within one year, cancer.

"He spent time with the Cancer Conqueror, who helped him analyze his resentment. 'I'm so mad because I don't have a job,' he said. The Cancer Conqueror helped him realize a new truth—perhaps he didn't have a job *because* he was so mad. He had to grasp his real need. For years he had harbored resentment. It was time to change—not just jobs, but some deep emotions."

The man listened intently as Barbara continued.

Our
Emotions
Don't
So Much
Happen
To Us;

We
Choose
Them.

"It's tough to deal with those emotions. They are at the heart of where we live every day. Just remember that our emotions don't so much happen to us; we choose them."

"That's an odd thought," said the man.

"At first it may seem odd, but examine it. When my husband and I went through our divorce, I was the classic victim. Then cancer. The illness merely reinforced my victim stance. I became a servant of my fears, angers, and guilts. I *chose* negative emotions.

"It wasn't until the Cancer Conqueror helped me reframe these negative emotions and taught me forgiveness that I was able to realize I could actually determine my own emotions. I realized I wasn't a captive of my fear, anger, and guilt—instead I was, or at least could choose to be, a product of love, joy, and peace.

"For the first time, I realized that we can't control life but we can control our *response* to life. And I also saw cancer as a message—as negative feedback—that up to now, I had not been making all the right choices. I changed. I chose life. I chose to LIVE!"

The man remained silent, deep in thought.

Barbara paused for a moment and when the man was ready, she continued, "It all brings us back to the core of resolve—the changing of our emotional lifestyles. By doing that, we prepare the body to heal. Clearing our lives of emotional difficulty is a LIVE message. This is resolving!"

"It's interesting," said the man. "Resolve isn't changing the circumstances so much as changing ourselves."

"Precisely," said Barbara. "We can't ever change anyone but ourselves. That is the key. It's true. I became a cancer conqueror not because I went into remission—instead, I became a cancer conqueror because I chose to become a new person!"

Another pause. More reflection.

You Become A
Cancer Conqueror
Not Because
You Go Into
Remission —

Instead,
You Become A
Cancer Conqueror
Because You Choose
To Become
A New Person!

"It all sounds so easy," said the man.

Barbara smiled, "Nobody will tell you it is easy. Simple? Yes. Easy? No. Just try to remember that change, like our emotions, is a choice. New choices are not easy. Pain is inevitable, but suffering is optional."

"Oh, that's good," said the man. "That's an excellent perspective. But how do I actually *do* all this? How do I make these changes real for me?"

Barbara reached for a piece of paper and began writing. "Here is the name and telephone number of a fellow journeyer. John has a whole new and exciting message for you to consider. And it is all centered on how to make these concepts work in your life. Call him and set up an appointment after you have begun to work through some of the resolve principles."

"I will," promised the man. "But before we quit today, will you help me summarize the principles we covered under resolve?"

"Of course," said Barbara. "Let's make a list."

RESOLVE SUMMARY

1. Emotions affect us physically.
2. Beliefs, attitudes, and feelings lead to illness or wellness.
3. Fear, anger, and guilt can depress the immune system.
4. The StresSolverSystem: I increase my personal power and decrease my problem power.
5. Hope and hopelessness are both a choice. Why not choose hope?
6. Instead of choosing to be a victim, I can choose to be a victor.

7. Cancer is a reversible disease.
8. My job is to forgive—myself and others.
9. Our emotions don't so much happen to us; we choose them.
10. You become a cancer conqueror not because you go into remission—instead, you become a cancer conqueror because you choose to become a new person!

SECTION 5

The Cancer Conqueror LIVES

The man spent an uncomfortable week trying to deal with the issues of resolve. It proved to be no easy task. And the man also had to admit he did not fully appreciate having to work on emotional conflicts. *It gets you in touch with some heavy issues. Aren't these things best left buried?* he thought. This was tough and frightening as well.

The man made a lunch appointment with John to talk about LIVE. Perhaps this would be an easier assignment. Maybe John would be able to help him through the difficult process of changing.

The man arrived at John's offices early. The receptionist pointed to an open double door and said; "You'll find him right in there. Go in."

As the man entered, he saw John not behind his desk but standing in front of it juggling three balls. "Come in," smiled John as soon as he saw the man. "Let's see how long I can keep these up!"

John's personality immediately drew a stranger in. Along with it came a big, easy smile and a nonpresumptive manner. Yet John's clothes, his grooming, and his posture also commanded a certain respect for this unusual businessman. Here was someone you liked and wanted to know more about.

"Oops!" laughed John as one of the balls dropped to

the floor. "I'm going to practice more tomorrow! Hello! Welcome!" he smiled as they shook hands.

John's deep voice was melodious. "I've had some fruit brought in for us," he said as he gestured to the conference table. "Let's just eat right here. Make yourself at home."

After only a couple of minutes of pleasantries, John said, "You impress me as a person of much intelligence. And because of that, I am going to take a chance. I'm first going to tell you a story that I believe will help you always to recall the central point of LIVE."

"Okay," chuckled the man, "go ahead." You just had to like John. His directness was refreshing and nonoffensive. Besides, how could you fault somebody who had already noticed your intelligence—someone who must be a keen observer of human talent? No doubt about it, John was joyful. He smiled as he began his story.

"Once upon a time there was a handsome prince.

"One day this handsome prince was on a walk in the forest when he met a wicked witch.

"The mean, old, wicked witch was very evil. She waved her magic wand and turned the handsome prince into a frog.

"As the wicked witch was leaving the forest, she said, 'The only way this spell can be broken is with a kiss from a beautiful fair maiden.'"

John continued, the big smile widening across his face. He was having fun!

"One day a beautiful fair maiden came to the edge of the stream where the prince-disguised-as-frog lived. Seeing his chance, he spoke to the beautiful fair maiden, telling her of his plight. 'And as the wicked witch left,' he finished, 'she told me that the only way the spell could be broken would be by a kiss from a beautiful fair maiden. Will you kiss me and turn me back into a prince?'

"The princess looked at him. Certainly she didn't *feel* like kissing a frog. How could she really know if he were telling the truth? In fact, this was preposterous. Who had ever heard of a prince disguised as a frog? And even if there should be a prince under there, why was she the one who had to give the kiss? It was a lot safer not to get involved.

"But then the princess began to consider the situation more carefully—*what if there really were a handsome prince under all that ugly green skin? What if he really were telling the truth? Just because she had never encountered this before did not mean that it wasn't possible. And why not she to be the deliverer of the kiss? It might actually be exciting to be involved, a whole new adventure.*"

John laughed as he continued, "What did she do? She took a chance! She trusted her positive instincts. She kissed that frog, and the handsome prince appeared. And they lived happily ever after."

John was smiling. "Now," he chuckled, "I go through that whole story for this one reason. And that is so you will remember that our job is to become frog-kissers!"

John leaned back and smiled broadly. The man had to smile, too.

"A frog-kisser? What does that mean?"

"What do you think it means?" asked John.

"I haven't the slightest idea," replied the man candidly.

John looked at the man. "What we are talking about, my friend, is love—nonjudgmental, unconditional love. And the truth is, that kind of love conquers cancer!"

"Love?" asked the man. "Is that where the journey leads?"

"It certainly does," said John. "It's what frog-kissing is all about."

"What do you mean?" said the man.

"If I could give you just one piece of advice on how to

Nonjudgmental,
Unconditional
Love
Conquers
Cancer.

conquer cancer," said John, "it would be to love, to be a frog-kisser. And my advice would be to love yourself first—to kiss the frog in the mirror.

"The Cancer Conqueror teaches that many people, particularly many cancer patients, grow up with the idea that they are somehow flawed and that this lack of perfection in some way makes them unacceptable. People who feel like this often act as if they must cover up this central defect if they are to be accepted, if they are to have any chance for love.

"Feeling unloved and feeling as if they are not worthy of love, these people, to greater and lesser degrees, retreat into isolation and loneliness. This retreat is a natural outcome of hiding their fear of another person's discovering that inner deficiency that makes them feel so unworthy.

"The Cancer Conqueror cites how often cancer patients tend to be perfectionistic, overachieving workaholics who repress their real feelings. They judge themselves by their work—how well they did it, how much they did of it, and how long they worked at it. And these same people often don't feel good about their accomplishments. They may even resent others for not noticing their work."

The man raised his hand to stop John. "That's me, a perfectionistic, overachieving workaholic! And nobody *ever* appreciates what I've done!"

"There are some heavy prices for living life by those beliefs," said John. "It's back to that whole thought of a central defect again. These people want to be judged by what they *do*—their work—rather than who they are as a person. And the trouble is, their good work is never good enough. And the praise, from self and others, is never quite loud enough!"

"Oh wow!" exclaimed the man. "You've just described me."

"Does this behavior often lead you to feelings of emptiness and disappointment?" asked John.

"Constantly," he nodded.

"Because of the profound inner emptiness and the despair, people with this characteristic often come to view
all their relationships in terms of finding something to fill
the void. This is the conditional love you hear so much
about. These people give love, give of themselves, give
anything, only on the condition that they get something
in return for it."

"Like what?" asked the man.

"It could be anything. People's conditions for love can
be vastly different. Some people want economic security.
Others want love and nurturing in return. Many people
seek approval from others. But there are patterns, a few
common threads running through each one.

"The trouble with behavior that places conditions on
love is that it is manipulative. It is conditional, contingent
upon getting something back. It is an 'if' love. It leads to
an even deeper sense of emptiness because it will always
fail."

"If the conditions are being met, it wouldn't fail. It
would work just fine," contended the man.

"Not for long," insisted John. "We're talking about human beings, people with expectations that escalate. It is
just a matter of time before either the expectations are not
met, or the people trying to fulfill those expectations
come to see themselves as being manipulated and quit.
But that's only the first level.

"On a deeper level, this 'if love' prevents the person
from understanding his or her true and unique self. If you
are always spending energy determining the degree to
which your expectations are being met, and the degree of
love which you will return, you'll never be able to understand the *true you*. You'll never be able to hear your own

music. It is a vicious circle that results in perpetual disappointment, deepening emptiness, and personal despair."

"Are you saying that I love conditionally?" asked the man.

"Yes. I do, you do, we all do," answered John. "At sometime in our life, we all love with 'ifs.' The trouble is, it doesn't stop there. That despair born of loneliness often leads to something even more insidious—judgmentalism.

"These are the ones who are consistently critical of people and circumstances that are different from their own views. The Cancer Conqueror points out that many people were brought up with a lot of 'shoulds,' 'oughts,' and 'have-tos': *A woman should be at home. A man ought to be a good provider. Children have to eat all their dinner.* There are literally hundreds of these learned rules.

"Those who are judgmental get into a pattern where other people's worth is measured by how closely they conform to the judgmental person's rules.

"Everything gets judged. Everyone is labeled as flawed and no good. All this is an attempt on the part of the judgmental to build themselves up while tearing others down. The vicious circle continues—disappointment, emptiness, and despair."

"This is really depressing," said the man. "I thought we were going to talk about LIVE."

John smiled, "We are. We're going to talk about how to LIVE by loving. But to do that, we need this perspective on judgmental and conditional love. The Cancer Conqueror once traced how crucial unconditional love really is. He believes that all disease has a lack of love as its roots.

"He explained how love that is judgmental and conditional leads to depression and thus allows physical vulnerability. He even went so far as to say that he felt all

Healing
Has At
Its Roots
The Ability
To Give
And
Receive
Nonjudgmental,
Unconditional
Love.

healing has at its roots the ability to give and receive nonjudgmental, unconditional love."

"What does this mean?" asked the man.

"It means that our task becomes learning to give and receive nonjudgmental, unconditional love. It means to stop judging. The Cancer Conqueror put this in an unforgettable, clear perspective when he talked about three valid standards to judge by. He feels there are moral standards, legal standards, and law-of-nature standards.

"Perhaps an example would help. Let's say friends with whom you have an appointment are late. Your reaction includes thoughts of anger. 'They don't respect my time. They are always late. They make me mad. They're really not considerate people.' There is a lot of judging going on here.

"But there is another choice. We could re-evaluate our thoughts about the lateness in light of the three standards. Does their lateness break any moral law? Is this in the same class as murdering someone or intentionally harming someone? Does their lateness break any legal standard? Is this behavior in the same class as speeding at a hundred miles per hour? And does the friend's lateness go against any natural law? Is the behavior in the same category as chlorofluorocarbons damaging the ozone?"

"Okay," chuckled the man. "Those are pretty exaggerated examples."

"Not really. Those are just the type of thoughts that trigger judging all the time. The point is that if someone's behavior doesn't break a moral, legal, or natural law, forget it! Don't judge it! If we can just release ourselves from judgmental behavior, we'll be a long way down the road toward learning how to love. And when we add unconditional love—loving without expecting anything in return—to nonjudgmental behavior, the two work together to form a powerful basis for living.

"I am convinced that the energy we have put into judging and into expectations can be redirected to help us get well. In that sense, unconditional, nonjudgmental love is a powerful stimulant to our natural immune systems. In that sense, love is not merely emotional. It is physiological. In a real sense, love can always conquer cancer and often cures it, too!"

John stopped as the man finished his notes. "It all relates to another facet of frog-kissing, acceptance versus approval. It's the difference between accepting people for who they are versus approving of them for what they do, their behavior. This applies not only to how you relate to others, but it especially applies to how you see yourself.

"For example, you must keep in mind that you are more than your behavior. You have great worth *outside* your behavior. You have worth as a person, as a living human being in addition to what you may do and even in spite of what you may do! The key is to truly learn to accept your worth as a person even though you may not approve of your behavior."

The man was silent, deep in thought. Finally, in a whisper, he said, "Tell me more."

"Okay," said John, "let's go from looking within to looking without. Let's examine other people. They are just the same as you and me. Their worth isn't wrapped up in what they do. We can learn to accept others as fellow citizens of the world even though we may not approve of their behavior. My task is to *accept* others, not *approve* of others."

"Accepting and not approving removes me from having to be the judge, doesn't it?" asked the man.

"That's it," John agreed enthusiastically. "That's precisely it. See, when we judge, we don't really see the other person, or ourselves, as whole people. Most of us were brought up in an environment where the emphasis was

*My Task
Is To
Accept
Others,*

*Not
Approve
Of Others.*

placed on constructive criticism. This is usually a disguise
for faultfinding. When we judge, we find fault and then
almost invariably label that person, or ourselves, as unworthy. We assume the other person to be wholly bad. We
assume ourselves to be wholly unworthy.

"But if we can separate persons from their behavior,
there is much to lovingly accept. We can go from being
faultfinders to becoming lovefinders! Only then can we
hear that strong inner voice saying, 'I love you and accept
you just as you are.'"

The man was again silent. This was new. And some-
what frightening.

If you decided to love, you left yourself vulnerable.
People could take advantage of that love.

"Can't other people take advantage of that love?" asked
the man, voicing his doubts. "Can't they take advantage
of you?"

"Only if you have expectations about extending that
love," said John. "Remember, our job is to love uncondi-
tionally. The person's reaction makes little difference.

"Perhaps the classic example is the case of the diners
who go into a fashionable restaurant for dinner. They find
the service deplorable and the waitress unfriendly and
rude. Feeling angry and mistreated, the diners feel justi-
fied in their grievance and hostility and leave the waitress
no tip.

"Now let's replay the scene from the start. This time
let's assume that the patrons discover, just as they sit
down, that the husband of the waitress died two days
ago and that she has five children at home who are solely
dependent on her for support.

"This changes everything. The customers adopt a new
role that overlooks the behavior as threatening and sees
the waitress as fearful, recognizing that she is calling out
for love and acceptance. Their response accepts her as a

person without having to approve of her actions and behavior. Their attitude is now loving, a response which they demonstrate by leaving an extra large tip.

"Do you grasp this?" asked John. "The scene was the same in each case. The characters were the same. The place was the same. The words were the same. However, in the first scene, the events were seen through the window of approval, with conditional love. And in the second, they were seen through the window of acceptance—nonjudgmental, unconditional love.

"What changed was the patrons' role. Nothing else. They went from faultfinding to lovefinding. We can live life this way! We can conquer cancer this way!"

The man was reflective. "Is this . . . frog-kissing?" he asked.

"Wonderful!" shouted John. "You've got it! That's it!"

Again the man was quiet and thoughtful. The idea had many implications. "This extends to other areas of life, doesn't it?" asked the man.

"It surely does," smiled John. "Frog-kissing has unlimited applications! Some people feel they are *married* to a frog! Some think they *work* for a frog. Some people see everybody else in the world as a frog."

Both men laughed.

"But those are just the windows of approval, judgment, and expectation that guarantee we will never know the power of love. Realize that other people do not have to change for me to love them. Instead, *I* have to change for me to love them! Isn't that a revolutionary thought?"

John jumped to his feet and waved his arms, "Our first job is to go from faultfinder to lovefinder—of ourselves and of others. And only we can make that choice. It depends on us! It's within our control. Isn't that wonderful? Isn't that a happy, hopeful thought?"

The man smiled. You just had to feel joy to see John

Other People
Do Not Have
To Change
For
Me To Love
Them —

I Have To
Change
For
Me To
Love Them.

wave his arms exuberantly and talk about love in his pleasant big voice. And he had to admit, there *was* hope in this frog-kissing message. How refreshing—within us there was wholeness, not some central defect. And outside us there were others whom we could choose to accept even though we may not approve. We didn't have to judge everyone! Going from faultfinder to lovefinder—this was *good!*

"There's a happiness in this outlook, isn't there?" asked the man. "Frog-kissing leads to joy, doesn't it?"

"You're great!" said John. "I can see you're going to conquer your cancer because you're so open to these principles. You've already grasped the next step in LIVE—joy! With love there comes happiness. And with happiness, joy is possible.

"You know, inside each of us is a child—the good, non-manipulative, fun-loving, filled-with-joy little person who needs to be nourished. It is the belief of the Cancer Conqueror that most cancer patients don't nourish this inner child. And by not honoring the child's real needs, they may be contributing to their illness or inhibiting their recovery.

"I used to deny the needs of my child," said John. "I always felt that those needs were far behind me. After all, I had matured. I had grown. I didn't need to laugh and play. Or so I thought. Wow, was I wrong! My needs to honor my inner child are very strong. I'll bet you have that same need."

The man said, "I'm not sure what you're talking about. Tell me more."

"There are two parts of finding joy. The first is an attitude issue. To me, joy is giving life a big hug, embracing all the beauty and wonder and goodness there is in this world. Joy is not how much you possess, but how much you enjoy.

Joy
Is Not
How Much
You Possess,

But
How Much
You
Enjoy.

"I once saw a bumper sticker that said, 'The one with the most toys wins!' My suggestion is that 'the one with the most *joys* wins.'

"It is that attitude that looks for joy in the small, precious packages and makes the most of them, knowing that the big packages of joy are really few and far between."

"That's joy!" said the man. "It sounds wonderful. I wish I were able to capture more of those moments."

"You can," said John. "You see, the second part of finding joy, of letting the inner child come out, is action. Simply put, we need to allow time for play."

"Play?" questioned the man.

"Yes, play," smiled John. "The kid inside needs time to play every day."

"But play sounds so . . . so . . . I guess it feels childish," said the man.

"That's the idea!" retorted John. "That's just what we're looking for—ways to nurture that inner child. This can really be an important step in your journey.

"The idea is to have fun, to create an enjoyable experience. The person who can find joy and laugh will be much better off than the stoic person who seldom cracks a smile and won't acknowledge his or her feelings.

"That's what you saw me doing as you walked in today. That juggling is one of my forms of play. And far from taking away from my capacity for work, it actually helps increase my energy for living.

"When I first heard the Cancer Conqueror talk about laughter and play, I, too, assumed it wasn't for me. I possessed a certain rigidity about releasing the inner child. Then the Cancer Conqueror talked about messages we may have learned as children. His ideas really hit home.

"Early on in life I was conditioned to 'try hard,' 'be serious,' 'be strong,' 'be successful,' 'be a good provider.' And I have heard women describe their messages of 'be

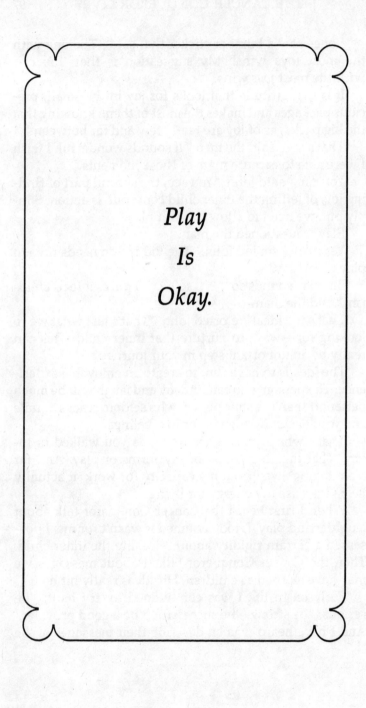

Play

Is

Okay.

perfect,' 'please everybody,' 'nurture everyone,' 'look nice.' When I realized how I had been conditioned, I actually had to start out by giving myself an assignment. I had to schedule time to play. Isn't that crazy?"

The man shook his head. "No, not at all. This cancer journey has once again confronted me with me. That's exactly the way I am. I learned the same things. I have the same attitudes toward play that you did."

"I hear you being a little tough on yourself," said John. "Instead, just decide to re-parent yourself on this one. First, I gave myself permission to play. I made play a more important part of my life. I used to say, 'I'll play after work.' Well, the work is never done. Now I let myself treat work and play with the same attitude—both are important. Both deserve my best. I had to decide that play is okay.

"The next thing I did was really helpful. I gave my inner child a name! As a youngster, nobody called me 'John.' I was known by my nickname, 'Buddy.' I always liked that. So I started calling my inner child 'Buddy'!

"It's great! I still do it! At first I asked what my inner child needed to *get* well. And today I ask Buddy what he needs to *stay* well.

"A helpful perspective for me was when the Cancer Conqueror suggested that we think of the part of us that got cancer as this inner child. Then our task becomes centered on taking care of that child, nurturing the child back to health, helping the child conquer cancer.

"So when I ask Buddy what he needs to stay well, I'm trying to get in touch with myself attitudinally, emotionally, and behaviorally on a very basic level. Buddy invariably wants me to honor his needs to experience laughter, play, and joy. And I listen. I now honor those needs," smiled John.

"That's neat how you talk with your inner child. I'm

What Does
My
Inner Child
Need
To Get
Well?

going to do that today!" said the man. "I've often sensed some of these things, but I never really talked to my child. This sounds exciting."

"When you talk to your inner child," said John, "you might want to do what the Cancer Conqueror suggests. He had me write out fifty different things I could do, actual activities I felt would bring me fun and produce joy in my life. Just try that exercise. It was very difficult for me to find fifty items at first. I suppose my child was so undernourished that he had forgotten how to play. But now my list has more than 150 activities—and it's still increasing."

"That's wonderful," said the man. "But I think I'm going to have trouble coming up with even ten ways to play."

"You'll learn," said John. "I found that it was important for me just to block the time to play. In the beginning there were some days that I didn't do a thing. But just scheduling the time, taking the time, was helpful. And soon I began to fill that time with activities.

"Once I heard the Cancer Conqueror talk about play in conjunction with treatments. A woman dreaded going in for treatments. So the Cancer Conqueror had her sandwich the treatments between play. Before she went in, she scheduled thirty minutes of piano playing for herself. And afterwards, she went window shopping, just to treat herself to the sights and senses there. Interesting. Her dread of the treatments decreased, and the side effects she was experiencing completely disappeared. She was now taking care of her inner child.

"So nurture your inner child," continued John. "Play is much more than an activity; it is an attitude that generates energy for healing. And we're never too tired to play. If we think that, perhaps that's a signal that we need play the most. Honor your inner child's needs."

"Thank you for giving me permission to do so," said the man. And he chuckled out loud. "You know, I already feel better. Just the idea of letting myself play is wonderful. And the idea of frog-kissing, maybe that's even better! I'm going to become a playful frog-kisser! How about that?"

Both men laughed out loud! Perhaps it was the mental picture that a playful frog-kisser conjured up. At any rate there was significant release in their laughter—a safety valve was being opened.

Then John spoke again. "It's wonderful to see you laugh, to see you smile and express that joy in your eyes. Yet as great as being a playful frog-kisser might be, there's something even better."

"What is it?" asked the man.

"Well, all the love in the world, all the joy in the world, resolving all our problems, even changing all our beliefs are empty without one essential ingredient.

"I once heard a person describe it this way, 'All our efforts are like a long string of zeros. They mean nothing without a digit in front of them. That digit is peace of mind.'"

The man was quiet, reflecting on what he had just heard.

"Inner peace is really the central message of the Cancer Conqueror. The goal is to have peace of mind, not just to cure cancer.

"Personal peace creates an environment conducive to healing within the body. It is perhaps the best way to allow the body's own healing mechanisms to function."

"Okay," said the man, "I like what you're saying, but really what is personal peace? And how do I go about achieving it?"

"Good questions," said John. "I like the definition the Cancer Conqueror teaches: 'Personal peace is

The Goal
Is To Have
Peace Of Mind —

Not
Just To
Cure Cancer.

transcending oneself in order to nurture inner harmony.'
Let's give this definition a closer look.

"First, personal peace is transcending. The idea is that
personal peace is intent, choice, and action. It is not some
chance occurrence. And personal peace transcends self—
meaning that the decision is made to consciously set aside
self-limitations of fear, anger, and guilt and to reach
for the serene greatness that rests within each of us. And
peace of mind is inner harmony, inner contentment, inner
tranquility. There is the definition. There is our goal."

"I don't hear you talking about outer quietness," said
the man.

"Many people would include that," said John, "and
others would not. For me, personal peace includes times
of outer quietness as well as times of activity. The Cancer
Conqueror really takes peace out of the activity realm
when he says, 'You will know personal peace when what
you think, what you say, and what you do are essentially
consistent.' I believe this is what we're really after—
inner consistency. Quietness may be a part of that. But
activity may also have a part.

"You see, it isn't so much the physical aspects as it is
the inner aspects, the emotional components, that make
for personal peace. This is especially important for the
cancer patient. Realize that peace of mind is independent
from our physical condition."

There was a pause. "Ah-ha," said the man. "A light
bulb has just gone on in my mind. Personal peace really
brings it all together, doesn't it?"

John nodded his agreement.

"How do I achieve this peace? How do I work to make
this a way of life?"

John stood, stretched, and walked across the office.
"You know," he began, "of all the changes the Cancer
Conqueror encouraged me to make, the daily pursuit of

*Peace
Of Mind
Is
Independent
From Our
Physical
Condition.*

personal peace has had the single most dramatic effect on my outer and inner life. If there were one change I had to point to which most altered my daily schedule, one which had the most potential for healing, it would be this pursuit—this acceptance of the profound personal peace that is available to all of us."

"I'm not sure I understand," said the man.

"I practice daily quiet time, a daily dose of tranquility, that gets me in touch with the deeper levels of personal peace that are always waiting there for me to enjoy."

The man looked a bit puzzled. "This seems a little far out. What do you mean?"

John smiled that reassuring grin as he sat down. "Just listen with your mind. There is so much healing potential here.

"Twice each day, I set aside fifteen minutes to calm my mind, to examine my spirit, and to affirm my total wellness in all areas of my life. Here at work, at home, when I travel, wherever I am, I find or make a quiet spot where I won't be disturbed. Twice each day—more if I am dealing with a lot of stress—I still my spirit, affirm myself, and find personal peace.

"I sit in a comfortable position, close my eyes and turn my attention to my muscles. I take special care first to tense and then to relax my muscles from head to feet, particularly those in the shoulder, neck, and forehead. In fact, one of my biggest muscle tension problems was my jaw—I was always clenching it, gritting my teeth, and pushing my tongue up against the roof of my mouth. No wonder I was always getting headaches. From the shoulders up, I was one knot of tense muscles. I now take time to consciously relax this area.

"Next, I conceive of my mind as the surface of a body of water. I have the mental picture of a lake. And when I think of the stress and tension that may have been part of my day, I see the surface of the lake churning with whitecaps.

"But then I imagine changing that scene, having the power to make those waves dissipate. I make the lake's undulating surface calm—placid and smooth, just like a mirror. At the same time I will repeat the word *peace* silently in time with my breathing.

"Amazingly, not only does my mind follow with thoughts that are calming and soothing, but my whole spirit feels a weight lifted. When a stressful thought or worry comes to mind, I gently dismiss it and make my thoughts go right back to the calm smooth surface of that lake and to my focus word *peace.*"

The man smiled, "I have to admit that just hearing you describe your daily dose of quiet is peaceful."

"Wonderful," said John. "That tells me you can easily and effectively do this exercise. Remember, the goal is first to relax the muscles. This, in itself, is a healing experience and will help in your total wellness. Then calm the mind. Dismiss thoughts that come and return to the placid, peaceful surface of the lake."

John continued, "I also use this as an opportunity to examine my spirit and to listen to the deeper messages of harmony found in quieting the mind. This relates to the resolve process.

"Many thoughts that cross my mind in my internal dialogue have to do with judging and with my feeling that I have to be right. When I observe my spirit and ask if those positions are bringing me love, peace, and joy, invariably it is a revealing and growing experience.

"I listen to my inner self. Some call this intuition. Others call it conscience, inner wisdom, or the subconscious. I just think of it as my inner self.

"I ask questions like, 'Am I experiencing love, joy, and peace?' Then I wait for my inner self to respond. 'Is my

marriage reflecting love, joy, and peace?' 'What about
my work? My physical condition? Our social life? Our
finances?' The idea is to examine the important areas of
life and then listen to the inner self evaluate.

"When I get a positive response, I'm thankful for it. I
express gratitude. When I hear a negative response, I ask,
'What is the message here? How do I need to change?'
Then I listen for direction from within.

"With practice, I was able to get on speaking terms
with myself. I now feel strong inner guidance is an important part of my life."

"How do you know you're not just selfishly coming up
with the answers you want to hear?" asked the man.

"Excellent question. You see, I truly believe that love,
joy, and peace are my aim and what is best for my life.
Love, joy, and peace are what is important. If I receive
signals that are based in fear, anger, and guilt, I know I
need to change. I need to let go again. If I receive answers
based on love, joy, and peace, I trust them because they
are consistent with my aim."

"But when you say, 'Let go,' what do you mean?" pondered the man.

"You've asked a profound question that has been
asked through the ages. To me," continued John, "letting
go means adopting an attitude of relaxed trust. Relaxed
trust is that sense of inner harmony—that serenity, that
contentment—which comes from knowing all is well,
even if you have cancer.

"You *can* let go. You don't have to judge. You don't
have to approve. You don't have to control. You don't
have to be right every time. You can give yourself a
vacation from trying to be Manager of the Universe!
That's letting go."

Both men laughed. How often they both had tried
to assume those roles and take those positions. New

thinking was required. "Examining, observing, listening—those are keys to a better way."

John continued, "And this leads to the final part of my daily quiet time—affirming myself. Many people use affirmations to replace old ingrained thinking patterns. Positive phrases, repeated often and with emotion, can lead to new understanding. They help counter conditioned thinking. Affirmations can help change our beliefs about cancer. The end of your quiet time is an appropriate time for these affirmations.

"But there is another side to affirming. This has to do with affirming—some would say directing, others might say rehearsing—your body's own built-in healing capabilities.

"The idea of mental reviews of desired activities is well accepted. Olympic athletes have used this creative imagination to gain a competitive edge. For example, the more an athlete imagines a successful jump over the crossbar, the more deeply etched the mental and emotional circuits become. In short, we become what we think about."

"Exactly what are you suggesting?" questioned the man.

John looked the man squarely in the eyes. "I am suggesting that you have significant control over your immune system, your natural defense against cancer."

"Is this more of the psychoneuroimmunology I have previously learned about?" asked the man.

"It is," said John. "And the primary technique for purposely stimulating our immune system is using creative imagination during our daily quiet time.

"One researcher called it healing with brain chemistry. Our immune defenses tend to weaken under stress. Quiet time with relaxation exercises and creative imagination may be one way to control the bio-chemical stress triggers and thus keep our resistance up."

"Do I hear you saying that in addition to my emotions influencing my immune system, I can also consciously enhance the functioning of my immune system?"

John spoke firmly and with deep conviction, "I am saying that creatively and consciously imagining our immune system functioning effectively may indeed enhance it. I am also recognizing that the immune system may be positively triggered as the roadblocks of fear, anger, and guilt are replaced with love, joy, and peace. And I am suggesting that as we imagine malignant cells being eliminated, and as we imagine ourselves as healthy, whole and feeling well, our entire being—body, mind, and spirit—will move in the direction of health. That is something we cherish! That is what we're striving for!"

"I've heard of this before," said the man. "In fact, I'm afraid I recently read that some doctors think the whole thing is self-deception."

"I'm sorry you read that," said John. "Instead of taking that article at face value, would you try an experiment with me here and now? Would you be willing to see if we could get our thoughts to trigger a system in our body?"

"Sure, I'm willing to do that. What do we do?"

John got comfortable, reclining slightly in his chair and stretching his legs out. He invited the man to do the same. "Okay, now just close your eyes and imagine yourself in your kitchen. Go over to the refrigerator and take out a big, yellow lemon that is in there. As you hold the bright, firm lemon, feel the texture of its skin. Feel the shape. See the color. Lift it to your nose and smell its sharp pungent odor. Now walk over to the counter where you find a paring knife. Cut the lemon in half. Notice the spray and smell the aroma as the juice runs over your fingers. Now take one of the halves and put it between your teeth. Bite hard and savor the juices as they roll over your tongue and throughout your mouth."

"Okay! Okay!" laughed the man. "You've made your point. I can't believe the amount of saliva that produces!"

"The fact is," said John, "the body cannot tell the difference between what is actually taking place and what you are *imagining* is taking place. This principle is at the very heart of what I was saying about the vital importance of imagining our immune systems functioning effectively. Does this example do anything to shift your thinking about this being some sort of deception?"

"Well, I have visualized many times before. I used it in my work. I know it works there. And I see no reason why it wouldn't work here."

John smiled. "That's it. You see, we have to protect our belief. Just one article that is negative, particularly if it is written by some authority figure like a doctor, can close the door on all sorts of possibilities. Let's learn to honor our own beliefs and respond to our own judgment."

"How did you go about enhancing your immune system?" said the man.

"My method was to see my cancer as something weak, and my immune system as something strong that would easily have the ability to handle the cancer. And during my treatment period, I imagined the chemotherapy as strong, a strong friend who was there to help rid my body of cancer."

"Yes, but how did you know what a cancer cell looks like? And the same for your immune system and the treatment?"

John gave a chuckle before he began. "You know what I did? I gave them all symbols. I didn't actually know what they technically looked like. I was told that wasn't important. It wasn't even critical that I knew where the cancer was located. What was important is that I imagined my immune system and treatment as being effective.

"So I imagined my cancer as ice cubes. And I saw my immune system as hot water. I viewed chemotherapy as an intense ray of white-hot light. The hot water and the ray of light melted the ice and the cancer was flushed from my body naturally. I felt this was a very effective image for me. Others have used the Pac-man game as something powerful for an immune system image. Still others that are frequently used include big fish that eat smaller fish, soldiers that defeat a weak opponent, or images of a similar nature.

"Just choose a weak image for the cancer and strong images for both your immune system and your treatment. And 'see' the dead cancer cells flushed from the body normally and naturally. Then end your quiet time by affirming yourself as healthy and free from cancer.

"This isn't self-deception. It is self-direction. And it moves us in the direction of wellness. What do you think about using your creative imagination?" asked John.

"Well, I think it is something I'm going to try. I can't help but believe in its potential. I've seen the principle work in other areas of my life. So I'm going to put it to use here."

"There's one more important thing that needs to be said," John added. "Creative imagination and affirming our own healing capabilities are different from quieting our minds and examining our spirits. Creative imagination is goal-directed. We actively guide our imagination. Quieting our minds and examining our spirits are observation-directed. They help us become more aware of thoughts and choices. They aid us in deciding to let go of those things that hold us back."

"Which is more important?" asked the man.

"Realize that we aren't simply imagining white blood cells attacking cancer cells. Instead, we are moving our entire being—body, mind, and spirit—in the direction of

We Are
Moving
Our Entire Being—
Body, Mind, and Spirit—
In The Direction
Of Wellness.

wellness. And this is a direction demonstrated by love, joy, and peace.

"I am suggesting that as important as your creative imagination can be, consider it as an adjunct to the main purpose of your daily quiet times. I suggest that you keep as your main goals quieting the mind and examining the spirit. The new awareness that they can bring is really what you are after. They generate peace of mind!"

The man finished his notes. "We've covered a lot of material."

John smiled that special smile once again.

"We have! But that's it, my friend. That's LIVE. Love, joy, and peace. To be a peaceful, playful frog-kisser! That's the goal. And it's also the essence of health!"

"That's a lot," said the man. "Can you help me summarize the points before I leave?"

"You've taken good notes," said John. "You can review them on your own. But write this down. It's the Cancer Conqueror's one sentence summary of LIVE:

To LIVE means to move our lives toward our own unique experience of love, joy, and peace.

"Spend time contemplating the special meaning of that for you."

The men stood. John put his hands on the man's shoulders and looked straight into his eyes. "Now go and live your life one day at a time. You can never tell when the greatest moment of your life is going to happen to you. So go and live each moment as if it were the greatest—the greatest for love, for joy, and for peace."

The men embraced. "Thank you," said the man. He left feeling at peace with himself and the world.

As soon as the man was home, he sat at his desk and summarized his notes.

LIVE SUMMARY

1. Nonjudgmental, unconditional love conquers cancer.
2. Healing has at its roots the ability to give and receive nonjudgmental, unconditional love.
3. My task is to accept others, not approve of others.
4. Other people do not have to change for me to love them; I have to change for me to love them.
5. Joy is not how much you possess, but how much you enjoy.
6. Play is okay. Make my list of fifty activities that are fun, that bring me joy.
7. Recognize and talk to my inner child. Ask, "What do you need to get well?"
8. The goal is to have peace of mind, not just to cure cancer. Peace of mind creates an environment conducive to healing the body.
9. Peace of mind is independent from my physical condition.
10. Schedule daily quiet time—at least fifteen minutes twice a day.
    — focus thoughts on a peaceful scene, dismissing other thoughts as they come and returning to that peaceful place.
    — listen to my inner self, being thankful for love, joy, and peace and being open to messages to change.
    — affirm myself and affirm my own immune system working to overcome the cancer.

SECTION 6

The Cancer Conqueror Explains

*T*he man felt good. John's LIVE message had given him hope! He called the Cancer Conqueror the very next morning.

"I have completed the assignment," he said. They scheduled a meeting that afternoon, right after the man's appointment with his doctor.

When the man arrived at the Cancer Conqueror's home, his mood had changed. The Cancer Conqueror picked up on the change immediately. "Compared to our phone call this morning, you seem troubled. Do you need to talk?"

"Yes, I do, and I'll tell you exactly what it is," said the man. I've just come from my oncologist's office. And while I'm doing great, just seeing all those patients in that waiting room wasn't a good experience. It's depressing! I talked with a woman who had just had a recurrence. It's a frightening prospect to work at getting well only to have the cancer return."

"Wait! Slow down!" said the Cancer Conqueror. "You're *awfulizing*, you're letting your thoughts assume the worst possible outcomes.

"Admittedly, an oncology office is not the best place to seek a lift. You see people there who are hurting, who are feeling hopeless and overwhelmed. When I need to schedule an appointment with my oncologist, I first become aware that I'll need to toughen myself mentally. And one of the issues is the people in that waiting room. I'm probably going to see some emaciated folks with fear and depression written all over their faces. Just looking at them can cause me to question myself and my own beliefs.

"But realizing this is helpful. If I am feeling strong emotionally, I often make an effort to sit by someone who looks especially needy. My goal is then to give whatever word of encouragement I can honestly muster. I try to take a negative and turn it into something positive. And when I do, invariably I feel better for having done so."

"Okay," said the man. "I understand what you're suggesting. But the fact is, I talked to a woman who had been cancer-free for seven years. Now it is back! The idea of a recurrence always haunting me is really frightening."

The Cancer Conqueror was firm. "The fact is, the possibility of recurrence will always be with you. The course of the disease is uncertain. Even so, there is reason for hope.

"There is a pervasive belief that is behind almost all worries of recurrence. The belief goes something like, 'Yes, you may battle the cancer with some success, but in the end the biological process will win and it will eventually get you.' Have you ever heard that?"

"Sure, just today I heard that from the woman who had the recurrence."

"That belief is a major untruth. It is reasonably common for people to go into remission, have a recurrence, and eventually enjoy recovery. Once again, the importance of our beliefs comes into play. We must first understand that recurrence does not mean imminent death.

"Yet, we need to treat recurrence as a crisis. For some, this is obvious. Their pain is significant, or perhaps they can actually feel growth. And it is common for fear to be

Recurrence
Does Not
Mean
Imminent
Death.

more intense with recurrence. They may also feel out of
control and lose faith in their medical team, their treatment, as well as the program they have been studying.
Feelings like 'I've failed; I give up' are common. That's
probably what you saw this morning with that lady."

"That was precisely it," said the man. "And it scares
me."

"I've gone through recurrence," said the Cancer Conqueror. "It was frightening. But I did some things that
made it a turning point. Consider these. First, I treated
myself very gently. I had been back at work, but now I
took more time off. I scheduled a vacation at one of our
favorite places. And I spent time alone, time to reflect.

"I talked with others, people who had overcome the
illness. It was helpful to understand that most of them
had also gone through recurrence. Almost all had used
recurrence as a time to reevaluate.

"So I followed their advice. I went back to the medical
team and had the doctors review the recent evaluations
in detail and answer my questions. This helped.

"Then I went back over my beliefs, examined the major
emotional stresses I needed to resolve, and looked more
closely at what personal needs weren't being met.

"Finally, I asked a tough question of myself. Did I want
to work toward health once again or did I want to accept
death and spend my energy preparing for it?

"You can see which I chose—I was willing once again
to work toward recovery."

"But what if you had died? There weren't any guarantees that you would recover," said the man.

"Not one," said the Cancer Conqueror. "But guarantees
aren't the issue. I said I would work toward recovery, that
I would work toward health. I couldn't guarantee recovery or health. No one could. I could only work toward
them. I had to realize that even though I didn't control

Even Though
I Don't
Control
My Destiny,

I Do
Influence
My Destiny.

my destiny, I did influence it. And I chose to influence it toward health."

The man finished his notes and looked up. "I need something with more certainty. I am expecting this program to bring me health."

"It can," said the Cancer Conqueror. "But are you also saying that you'll reject it if it doesn't meet all your expectations? I can't give you any guarantee. I can only share that for me it was—and is—a hill-and-valley experience.

"I refused to view the valley of recurrence as a failure. Instead, I again chose to view recurrence as a message. I needed once again to understand the message and decide what my response would be.

"For me the message of recurrence was clearly that I was not taking care of myself as I needed to. Up to that time, I was not really following the diet I knew was best for me, I was exercising only occasionally, I wasn't taking time to play, I only sporadically worked with my creative imagination, and I had only partially resolved some of the emotional conflict issues.

"When I honestly looked at myself, I realized that I had, in many ways, returned to the lifestyle that contributed to my initial illness. After I realized this, I came to believe that recurrence was my body's way of telling me to choose to change once again—to work toward health or to accept death and begin that process."

The man was uneasy. "Maybe the real issue of recurrence with me is the possibility that death is near. That scares me so much. I don't want to die. It's all so frightening."

"Okay," said the Cancer Conqueror. "Let's talk about death. When you think about death, what is it that you fear?"

"Oh, wow," said the man pensively. "The whole thing is frightening. I don't even like to think about it. Maybe it's the fear of lying there helpless, not being able to take care of myself. I don't want to be an invalid. And the people we leave behind. That's sad. And it's also this emptiness about no longer existing. I get depressed just thinking that it's all going to come to an end. I hate to talk about death."

"Then let's face this fear," said the Cancer Conqueror. "Instead of saying we don't want to deal with an issue, let's just take fear of death and start to conquer it right now.

"You said you feared three things about death. One was the issue of being an invalid. That has to do with the process of dying, the quality of death. And you also said you felt sad about leaving. That has to do with severing our earthly ties. Finally you said you felt empty about no longer existing. This is the issue of what may or may not come after death."

"Yes," sighed the man. "That's it."

"There is much we could say about death," said the Cancer Conqueror.

"Much has been written about it. I encourage you to seek out the resources you need to handle this issue. So today, let's not make it our aim to fully explore death. Instead, let's just attempt to help you through the basic issue of facing your own fear of death.

"I remember discussing the issue of death with a pastor. In a blinding flash of the obvious he said, 'First, I assume you believe you will die. I mean, the statistics are overwhelming! A thousand out of a thousand people die! There don't seem to be many exceptions! Life in that body will end someday.'

"The implications of his humor hit me immediately. Of course I would die. The question wasn't 'if'; the question was 'when' and 'how.'

"Many cancer patients are anxious about death's

'when' and 'how.' There is sadness and possibly anger over the prospect of a shortened life—the when. Perhaps there are dreams still to pursue and people still to love. So the thought of shortening the lifespan seems unfair.

"Yet in a real sense, people live on in the memories of others. If we want to guarantee a loving memory, if we want to guarantee that we accomplished something great with our lives, then we need to love, and love now! That's the secret to overcoming the fear of death's 'when'—it's to love now, today, this hour, while we have the opportunity. A life's value is not measured by its duration but by its donations of love!"

"That's helpful," said the man. "Very helpful."

"And then there is the dread of a low quality of death. A long, debilitating illness that could drain the family and the patient emotionally and financially is the real fear. This is the unpleasant 'how' part, a fear that there is little control over death.

"Unlike many causes of death, cancer usually allows ample time to prepare. This preparation, this taking control can be very comforting. Some may want to plan their funeral. Others may want to sign a living will which instructs doctors to discontinue life-support systems when there appears to be no hope of survival. Normally there is time to prepare wills and put estates in order.

"All these things can be done to gain some control over death. And there's even more control. It's amazing. A study of several thousand deaths showed that almost 50 percent occurred within three months after people's birthdays, while fewer than 10 percent came in the three months prior to their birthdays."

"I don't understand the point," said the man.

"Just this," said the Cancer Conqueror. "People seem to have an influence over the time of death. Many

A
Life's Value
Is Not
Measured
By Its
Duration

But
By Its
Donations
Of Love.

'postponed' their death until after they had celebrated their birthday."

"That's incredible," said the man. "Can we be certain?"

"No," said the Cancer Conqueror, "there isn't a certainty here. I'm not saying that we can live as long as we want. But I am suggesting that we do have some degree of control that perhaps we once thought did not exist."

The Cancer Conqueror continued, "And another point on control. I've been able to work with a team of professionals who, as part of a total cancer treatment plan, teach patients about death. The senior oncologist feels that there is strong evidence that many people die as they have lived."

"What does he mean?" asked the man.

"It's back again to this issue of fearing a low quality of death. He observes that patients who live a resentful life many times experience a 'resentful' death, full of prolonged suffering. And likewise, many patients who live a life of anger may experience an 'angry' death. But also, those who live a life of love, joy, and peace nearly always reflect this in their death.

"Again, the lesson here is to love. We can choose to love now, to be joyful now and to make peace of mind real now. In short, we can choose to 'live fully as long as we live' by showing love to ourselves and to those around us. The result in terms of quality of death is almost always a reflection of that way of life. Very little time is spent actually dying; the time is spent living and loving as long as we are alive."

"I like that," said the man as he took a moment to ponder the point.

The man seemed touched by the hope in the Cancer Conqueror's message. There was a comfort in understanding that he could control the quality of death by the quality of his life. And the idea of extending the reach

Choose
To Live
Fully
As Long
As We
Live!

of one's life through the memories of others—by loving others—was also reassuring.

But what about himself after death? Was he just a memory? That seemed less than fully satisfying.

"What about life after death?" asked the man. "Do you think there is more to come after this life?"

Without hesitation the Cancer Conqueror answered, "To me the evidence is overwhelming. I believe that you and I are much more than a body. I certainly do not pretend to know everything about this issue. Yet I believe very strongly that death is the exit from this life and the entrance to the next plane of existence. To me, death doesn't have to be approached with fear. I think we can approach it with a healthy curiosity of what will be next. It can be viewed as a new adventure. Can you grasp that possibility?"

The man was deep in thought. Finally he looked at the Cancer Conqueror and almost in a whisper asked, "There's comfort in those beliefs, isn't there?"

The Cancer Conqueror nodded, "For me there is. There's real comfort and real hope. I believe there is much that awaits me after life here on earth. But my concept of life, not death, is what makes the difference. This compels me to love now. The result is inner harmony and personal peace about whatever may be on the next plane."

The man stopped again. He was considering some of the implications of what the Cancer Conqueror was saying. "The next plane. Inner harmony. Personal peace. This almost has a mystical quality to it. Does the cancering journey become some sort of religious experience?"

"Some people would not be comfortable with the words *religious* or *mystical*. I prefer to use the term *spiritual* when we discuss this. And yes," said the Cancer Conqueror, "in my experience, cancering becomes very much a spiritual journey."

"Then please help me understand this part," said the man.

"Just consider the context," said the Cancer Conqueror. "We live in two worlds, the material and the spiritual. Most of our education, our efforts, even our awareness are centered in the material. But consider the cancer journey. While there is certainly a material, physical element, we move beyond that. We talk about beliefs—beliefs that are positive, that serve our health well. Then we move on to resolve, managing the emotional conflict that can depress our mind and our body's immune system. And then we make a choice, a conscious decision to LIVE. Those are all issues of the human spirit. The context becomes spiritual."

"John made that clear," said the man. "I understand the principles. But I sense I am missing a dimension. I sense this all leads somewhere."

"Excellent," said the Cancer Conqueror. "It certainly does lead somewhere. As you begin to choose the spiritual life, you'll also begin to recognize the breadth and depth of that choice. It pervades your entire life experience."

"That's good," said the man, "'. . . pervades your entire life experience.' I feel that's what is happening to me right now. I sense that I am beginning to open to a whole new life. What is actually going on here?"

The Cancer Conqueror deliberated a moment. Was the man ready for a more in-depth look at the spiritual road? Would he be able to grasp the dimensions of this choice? And could the Cancer Conqueror explain it in a way that would not alienate him? It was a tender moment. The Cancer Conqueror inched ahead.

"I can best explain this by starting once again with beliefs. This time the beliefs are not about the illness. They are about life.

"There are certain core convictions, foundational beliefs that profoundly affect our life experience in virtually every aspect. They do much to determine the quality of life on all levels. These beliefs—these core mental choices— affect us far beyond just our bodies, far beyond cancer."

"Okay," said the man, "what are they?"

"Perhaps the most fundamental belief has to do with the essence of the world in which we live. For centuries, the great thinkers have debated—what is the nature of the universe? Did biological accident or Divine direction create our experience? In short, the first core belief asks the question, 'Is there a God?'

"I encourage you to choose a healthy conviction here. I encourage you to believe that there is a God who knows us and loves us. And God loves us even though God knows us!"

"That's a healthy choice?" asked the man.

"Very healthy," said the Cancer Conqueror. "There are significant assumptions in that statement. First, there is the choice that God really does exist and that God lies behind our existence."

"Well, sometimes I'm not so sure," said the man.

The Cancer Conqueror smiled, "I can't offer you hard, scientific, rigorously researched and documented proof that there is a God. I can't take you down the street to a church and say, 'See, look at God.' On this point, trust in your beliefs is the determining factor."

"I don't know," said the man. "This is more than I am comfortable with."

The Cancer Conqueror touched the man's arm. "Look, the last thing I want to do is make you uncomfortable. But *I* am not the one who is making you uncomfortable. *You* are making you uncomfortable."

"Okay," said the man. "But the fact remains, I just don't know that much about God."

There Is
A God
Who Knows Us
And
Loves Us.

And
God Loves Us
Even Though God
Knows Us.

"You do know that there is something outside your-self, don't you?" asked the Cancer Conqueror. "After all, you didn't make this world. And I didn't create the universe. Certainly there must be some kind of Power outside of you and me. A Greater Power is behind our existence."

"Well, from that standpoint, there must be something," said the man.

"But does that mean 'God?'"

"Perhaps you're letting the word *God* get in your way. To some people the word *God* is full of negative connotations, especially that of judgmentalism.

"In all the languages of the world, people use different names for the Deity. The most widely used in the English language is *God.* For the moment, try to drop some of your previously learned concepts about God. Would you be able to explore the spiritual path openly just for a few minutes?"

"Okay," said the man. "I can do that."

"Good," said the Cancer Conqueror. "For the moment, just accept that there is 'something' that is a Higher Power. We call that power God. Let's look again at the core belief. There is a God who knows us and loves us, and God loves us even though God knows us.

"So there is a primary conclusion, an affirmation, a conviction that acknowledges a Power behind our existence. There is a God of the world."

The Cancer Conqueror continued, "The second part of our core belief states that there is a God 'who knows us.' The implications of this statement are significant. Not only are we saying that there is a God, but we are also believing that this God is aware of you and me as individuals. You are known to God personally, by name, by thought, by spirit, by all the ways that God can identify and recognize us. This is no abstract power—this is a personal one-on-one relationship with the Central Power behind everything that exists."

The man was thoughtful. Even though he didn't speak, the Cancer Conqueror could sense his attentiveness.

"Now take our core belief another step. The belief goes on to say '. . . and God loves us!' This thought is a revolution. Not only is there a God who knows us personally, but that same God *loves* us. The very Power that created everything that exists knows and loves us! Wow!"

The man smiled at the Cancer Conqueror's enthusiasm. But perhaps this was something to be enthusiastic about. It was certainly different. The man had always thought of God as some sort of mean judge.

The Cancer Conqueror continued, "Let's finish our look at the core belief. It ends by stating, '. . . and God loves us even though God knows us.' This means that even when we don't perform to our potential, we are still loved. In the eyes of the Creator of All, we are not what we do or don't do. We receive God's love simply because we are God's creation. God chooses to love us as we are!"

The man said, "But I don't see how this influences my cancer journey."

"All this acknowledges the fact that God is for us! God wants our total wellness. Our job is to get in tune with the messages cancer is sending us, make the required changes, and accept God's love and direction for our lives!"

The man snapped, "How can that be? If God is for us, why did God give us cancer?"

The Cancer Conqueror paused and smiled that serene smile. He understood how critical his next words would be. "I don't believe God did give us cancer," he said. "My belief is that this illness is not God's will, but is really the result of our deviation from God's will.

"In fact, I now believe that those things which bring

sorrow, distress, or even calamity and suffering are ultimately present in the world not as God's will, but as a
result of our misunderstanding or our deviation from
God's will."

"Well maybe," said the man, "but it seems to me that
God at least allowed the cancer."

"Perhaps," said the Cancer Conqueror. "But even that
is not the perspective you'll need to conquer cancer. The
key is to understand the message. It is really an opportunity for us to change. I've even thought of cancer as a
gift, a valuable opportunity to reshape my life. And
when I began to understand the depth of this, my whole
thinking about God and my life changed."

There was silence. The two men looked squarely into
each others' eyes. The man sat with clenched jaw, pondering the implications of what was being said. The Cancer Conqueror sent up a silent prayer, "Speak through me
now, Lord," and then continued.

"Understanding the meaning and message in cancer
brings us face to face with our second core belief. It has
to do with the nature of our life experiences. There are
many ways to say this. But the one which communicates
best to me says, 'Life is a loving teacher.'"

"If God loves us," continued the Cancer Conqueror,
"God will want the best for us. God will lovingly guide
and direct our paths. Thus through our life experiences—
both pleasant and unpleasant—lessons are going to be
taught."

"I have trouble believing that a God who is lovingly
trying to teach us would be so cruel as to cause or even
allow cancer. That's just not loving."

"Now think," continued the Cancer Conqueror firmly,
"of the consistency with the earlier belief that cancer is a
process and a message to change. Some lessons that God
lovingly gives, or even allows, are pleasant. Other lessons

Life
Is
A
Loving
Teacher.

are anything but pleasant. Yet both teach, guide, and direct our lives. Perhaps there are times when we get so off the track that the only way God can get our attention is through an event that is nearly catastrophic."

"This sounds like the vindictive, judge-type God that I was taught about as a child," said the man.

"Not so," countered the Cancer Conqueror. "God is not some unreasonable and impulsive sovereign. This is a loving God who has created a universe that runs by natural laws. This loving God doesn't give out punishment on a whim."

"But God is omnipotent," said the man. "God can do anything God wants to do."

"Certainly," said the Cancer Conqueror, "but also recognize that God has put in place the natural laws that run the world. And God seldom breaks those laws. They are the natural order of this world.

"It is healthy to believe that even cancer is a message for us to become more aligned with those natural laws. That is what life is trying to teach us—to become more aligned with God's will."

"That's hard for me to accept," said the man.

"Think of it this way, then," said the Cancer Conqueror. "Illness and health send us messages, negative and positive. Both messages tell us how we are doing. Health, happiness, peace, joy, and love are all intended as messages that we are doing well. Illness, pain—both physical and psychological—depression, fear, and despair are all negative messages that are intended to bring us back on course. They are all loving teachers."

The man shook his finger at the Cancer Conqueror. "But your logic is all wrong. The true nature of people is not good, it is evil. I can remember the exact words I was taught, '. . . man is by nature sinful and unclean.' It doesn't make sense to have a loving God who is a loving teacher if people are inherently bad. These lessons you talk about would never get through. You need to punish evil."

The Cancer Conqueror was dismayed. These were all learned beliefs and behavior—real roadblocks that had been constructed in the man's spiritual path. But they explained the man's behavior.

"No, no, no!" said the Cancer Conqueror. "Emphatically no! I don't like to confront you, but this is an important point. There is a better way. There are better beliefs! In fact, this is core belief number three—God created people in innocence and goodness.

"I went through this struggle," said the Cancer Conqueror. "I was taught that original sin had left me totally helpless, that some people are predestined to live in eternal despair and that my behavior could be controlled only with a heavy dose of fear and guilt. I was frightened by a God who I thought was out to get me.

"These beliefs are not true. They confuse what a person does with the way God originally created people. In point of fact, virtually all religions acknowledge that people were created in innocence and goodness. The concept of 'evil' we hear so many people emphasize came later.

"When the emphasis is on 'evil,' guilt almost always is the end result. This is sad and destructive. These teachings simply do not go deep enough. And worse, they inflict untold scars on people. It is my personal belief that many illnesses, including cancer, may be caused or prolonged because people condemn themselves and others with this guilt."

"I'm not sure what you're saying," said the man. "How does this apply to my getting well?"

The Cancer Conqueror continued, "Simply stated, if you believe either consciously or subconsciously that God created people as inherently evil, you will consider

God
Created
People
In
Innocence
And
Goodness.

yourself unworthy. And unworthiness certainly isn't a perspective of wellness."

"Well then," said the man, "what is that wellness perspective?"

"Let me encourage you to hold firmly to the conviction that people, at the very core of their being, have unlimited potential for kindness, goodness, and gentleness—particularly as they relate to God. Believe in people's ability to love. Perhaps the message behind cancer is that God can change us! Perhaps the real message of cancer is threefold: love God, love others, love ourselves."

"But there is so much evil out in the world. How can we say that people have the capacity for unlimited kindness, goodness, gentleness, and love? I think this is very much at odds with actual experience," said the man.

The Cancer Conqueror smiled. "Remember the central lesson of LIVE—nonjudgmental, unconditional love?"

"Yes I do," said the man. "It was a huge leap in personal growth for me. But how does it apply here?"

"Let's review," said the Cancer Conqueror. "First we looked within to realize that we do not have some terrible central flaw in our being that makes us hopeless. Next we looked without to realize that others were just the same and that we could learn to accept them as fellow human beings even though we may not approve of their behavior. And finally we saw our role—to be loving and forgiving without expecting to get something in return."

"Yes I know," said the man. "That liberated me. But I still don't see your point."

The Cancer Conqueror looked unwaveringly into the man's eyes. This would be a critical point for the man to grasp. He shot up another prayer for guidance.

"Just as you have been liberated by extending nonjudgmental, unconditional love to yourself and to others, know that a loving Gcd is extending even more and greater love to you."

The Cancer Conqueror paused for several seconds before he spoke again. "And even though our behavior may not always match our potential, even though our potential for kindness, goodness, and gentleness is not fully realized, we can receive God's love because God loves us for who we are, not for what we do!"

Another long pause. "Because of God's great love, we are still acceptable even though we may be imperfect." He repeated, "We are imperfect but acceptable."

The Cancer Conqueror just stopped and fixed his gaze directly on the man's eyes. The long silence was finally broken by the whisper of the man himself.

"Imperfect but acceptable."

The Cancer Conqueror didn't say a word. He just nodded his head in agreement. Tears welled up in the man's eyes. You could sense a transformation underway.

The man sunk back in his chair. "Nobody ever explained it like this before," he said ever so quietly. "A loving, personal God, the Creator of all there is, life as a loving teacher, and people who are not rejected because of their imperfections.

"I'm not perfect, but I am acceptable and I am loved," he continued in a hushed voice. "I can't tell you what this means to me." He paused again. "This is the first time in my life that I have received and experienced and appreciated nonjudgmental, unconditional love."

The man stopped speaking. It was an emotional moment of silence.

Finally the Cancer Conqueror spoke. "This is a love that heals. This love is the gateway to that peace we are accepting. This love ultimately conquers cancer. And the bonus is that this love often cures it, too."

More silence. The man was meditating. At last he

We Are
Imperfect—

But

Acceptable!

asked, "There are no guarantees on this path, are there?"

"If you're looking for a sure cure on the purely physical level, nobody can offer you one with integrity. But on the spiritual level, the answer is right before you. You are known. You are loved. You are acceptable. Yes. It's guaranteed."

The two sat quietly. The man felt a sense of peacefulness that was completely new to him.

"I want to know more about the love of God," said the man. "Where do I turn? Do I go back to church? Do I take up religion? Do I pray day and night? What do I do next?"

The Cancer Conqueror smiled. "You may personally feel you need to do one or even all these things. That will be your decision. But start with the inner journey. Start with aligning yourself with God's love. Practice God's unconditional love without ceasing."

"And then what?" asked the man. "What did you do?"

"When I became aware that God is my Source," said the Cancer Conqueror, "I turned to the God of the Scriptures. Here I discovered a special power that could be found nowhere else."

"This," said the man, "is the very point I have so much trouble with. Can I really believe? Can I really trust this God?"

"Yes, you can," said the Cancer Conqueror. "You can trust God completely. But, don't expect God to do it all for you.

"I want you to trust three physicians. *Trust the body physicians*, your medical team. Trust their competence and their integrity to do all they can for you on a physical basis. *Trust your inner physician*, the inherent ability you possess to generate emotional harmony and physical healing. And *trust the spiritual physician*, the God who loves you and gives you peace."

"Why not just pray for God to perform a miracle?" asked the man.

"God could," said the Cancer Conqueror. "We certainly want to allow for that. And God sometimes does that. But the natural laws that God governs by are seldom broken. Law-of-nature-defying miracles are certainly the exception. But law-of-nature-consistent miracles are happening everyday. They can happen to you.

"And God is not lessened because of that. Believing in our own healing potential only goes to acknowledge our true spiritual nature."

Both men were quiet as they let these insights saturate their spirits. There was power for living here. Finally the man said, "You know, I have a sense of calm, of real peace—right now. I've never experienced this before. This is a new me."

The Cancer Conqueror smiled. This was the place where he had hoped to bring the man.

"Peace is the goal," the Cancer Conqueror continued softly. "Knowing God's peace—even if we have cancer—that's what it really means to conquer the illness.

"Our goal is peace—with self, with others, with God. And that goal is achieved by implementing the very things you have studied—Believe, Resolve, and Live!

"When the goal of peace is achieved, it may be temporary. In fact, try not to relate peace to time at all. It may be difficult to achieve that peace for more than a few minutes. If so, don't be discouraged. It is the journey, not just the destination, that is the aim."

"I think I've heard that principle elsewhere," said the man. "Is that why everyone kept referring to the 'cancer journey?'"

"It is," said the Cancer Conqueror. "It is a journey in search of God's peace. And the sooner you make it a LIVE

Our Goal Is Peace —

With Self,
With Others,
With God.

journey, the sooner you will benefit from life's lessons—
and experience your own peace."

The Cancer Conqueror continued, "Now consider this.
If cancer is a message to change, what is it that you are
being called to be and to do? Put the emphasis here
on *called.*"

"What do you mean?" asked the man.

"Just this. Cancer is telling you to change. It's a call
toward a new goal and a new way. You are called to be
someone. You are called to do something. Pursue that
goal. Within it will be your reason for living.

"Don't be driven," continued the Cancer Conqueror.
"Be called. Take time to listen and respond to the call."

"That call," asked the man, "is it centered in loving and
helping others?"

"You know it is!" said the Cancer Conqueror. "Plus
responding to God's directions for your life. Your call
will take the form of love toward self, love toward others,
and love toward God. And you'll know you are succeed-
ing when what you think, what you say, and what you do
are consistent with God's directions."

Again the two men sat in silence. There was peace in
this silence. The Cancer Conqueror prayed. The man was
listening to that call from within.

Finally the Cancer Conqueror spoke. "The achieving is
in the doing. Go and do."

There was another silence. Finally the two men stood
and embraced. And then the man left silently. God's
peace was with him.

SECTION 7

The Cancer Conqueror Benefits

*A*s the weeks passed, the man put to use what he had learned. And guess what happened?

He became a Cancer Conqueror!

It happened not just because the man talked like a Cancer Conqueror, but because he had learned a better way to LIVE!

And as the weeks built into months, he realized that it was not simply that he had learned new skills and knowledge, but that he *did* what he had learned.

This *was* a better life. Cancer really *was* a signal to change. New freedom was his! Love, joy, and peace were real to him!

At the end of the first year, the man looked back to the day when he had first met the Cancer Conqueror. Since that time, he had changed so much. His beliefs about cancer were radically different. And he had begun to resolve some fundamental problems he hadn't even recognized prior to the cancer. And LIVE had given him freedom he had barely imagined.

The man was thrilled to understand for the first time in his life that he really was the one in control. But it was a control unlike the control that most people sought.

For certainly the man was not the Ultimate Power. Nor was he immune to all the problems life had to offer! But rather the man had developed a new power over himself, a power within, which allowed him to choose how to react to the events of life. He had begun to align himself with God's will. This is where the power and control came from. This was living! This was Conquering Cancer!

The man began sharing his own journey with newly-diagnosed patients. It was most encouraging to see people change their beliefs, resolve their difficulties, and then choose to LIVE!

The man made himself more and more available for these times of sharing. Cancer had taught him some valuable lessons. He was becoming a student of life. And at the same time, he was becoming a teacher of living.

He enjoyed helping others learn to help themselves.

Perhaps what he enjoyed most, though, was the mastery over his own life. Every day, in every way, he was learning to LIVE!

He felt capable of dealing with today in a way that helped others as he helped himself and the world in which he lived.

The phone rang.

A young woman introduced herself. She explained that she had just been diagnosed with cancer. "I have been told that I have a journey ahead of me. I know I have a lot to learn. I would like to learn from the best. May I come talk to you?"

The man smiled that serene smile he had seen so many times before. Now he realized the smile was a sign that all was well—*very* well!

It felt good to be in this position. He *had* learned a great deal. He was one of the most significant success stories because he had come from despair to hope. Now he knew inner peace—God's peace. It was a simple journey. But it had not been easy.

"Of course you can come talk with me," he answered.

As soon as the young woman arrived, he began the conversation. "I'm happy to share my experiences with you. In doing so, I have just one request."

"What is that?" she asked.

"That you share this hope with others!"

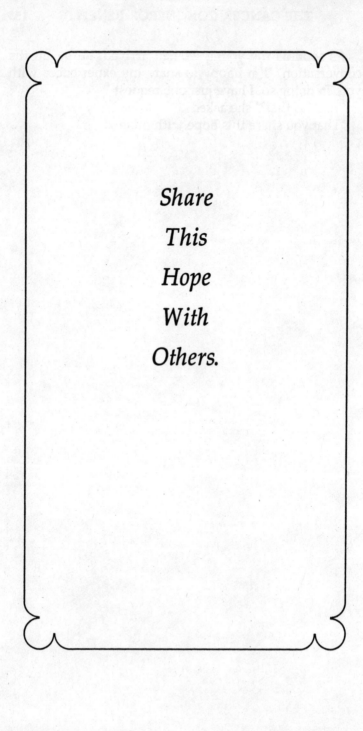

Share
This
Hope
With
Others.

EPILOGUE

Imperfect but acceptable.

For some of you who read this book, you came face to face with unconditional love for the first time. Its meaning may be liberating to you. For others, you may recognize the love. Its meaning to you may call for surrender. And for still others, this book means coming to a decision regarding an initial commitment to that unconditional love. I call this Unconditional Love Jesus Christ.

God's love for you is fully reflected in His spiritual gift to the world—His Son, Jesus Christ. Jesus is the epitome of Unconditional Love. Unfortunately, throughout history some of His followers have filled the path of love with ecclesiastical roadblocks and stained-glass barriers. See through those. Be nonjudgmental to these people. Keep your focus on God and His loving Son, Jesus.

All of us know now is the time to act. Some of you are showing great resistance to aligning your will with God's will for your life, and you know it. But you can't dodge the issue any longer.

Talk to Christ now. There is no need for fear. Jesus sees you as acceptable! Then just listen as God speaks to you.

All His best,
Greg Anderson

ABOUT THE AUTHOR

Greg Anderson is a Cancer Conqueror. Diagnosed with metastasized lung cancer, Anderson was given only thirty days to live. Refusing to accept the hopelessness of this diagnosis, he went in search of others who had lived when they were "supposed" to die. His incredible findings form the principles in this powerful book.

Today, Greg Anderson is Founder and President of Cancer Conquerors, an educational and support group that teaches cancer patients and their familes how to integrate body, mind, and spirit. He is the former Vice President and Executive Director of the Robert Schuller Institute located at the Crystal Cathedral in Garden Grove, CA.

SERVICES AVAILABLE

Cancer Conquerors was conceived because of the increasing demand for body/mind/spirit education in the United States and abroad. The organization provides training for both patients and their families. These services include seminars of one to five days, instruments for self-assessment, audio and video programs, training internships, and ongoing personal consultation. The group's goal is to help its members facilitate life healing in all its dimensions.

For further information please write:

Cancer Conquerors
P.O. Box 3444
Fullerton, CA 92634